Dis-ease
To
Ease

Healing across 4 Dimensions
from periphery to the core

Saleem Anwar

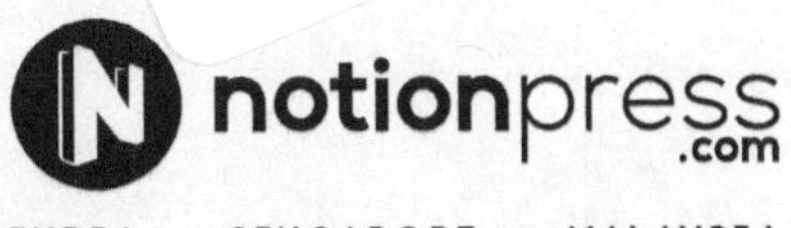

ISBN
Paperback 979-8-89699-530-2
Hardcase 979-8-89777-319-0

"Know what sort of person has a Disease rather than what sort of Disease a person has"

– Hippocrates

CONTENTS

PROLOGUE

One day, God said to the Angels. "I'm going to place my representative on Earth."

"What? Even while we are obedient and diligent in our duties?" the Angels questioned.

God replied, "That is the problem—your obedience. I want a being with free will, someone who can co-create with me, **cautiously**, my way. I am power personified, yet I channel my power to create this magnificent universe and all it holds."

The Angels were puzzled: "But you are One, unique, and they would be many. Wouldn't it lead to chaos and bloodshed as each looks to create according to their whims and fancies?"

"There is a check," God responded. "When their will aligns with mine, and they work selflessly, there will be Peace, Bliss, and Harmony—a state of Ease, Heaven. But when they misuse their freedom, choosing selfishness and excess, they will sow discord and find themselves in a state of Disease - Hell."

The Angels asked, "Is there no way back for them, God?"

"There is," God assured them. "The moment they realize their folly and ascend the evolutionary ladder by cultivating just one sublime attribute of mine—**Compassion**—they will regain their lost Paradise, the State of Ease."

The word "compassion" here is a loose translation of the Arabic *Rehman*. Unlike its Latin root *compati*, meaning "to suffer with," in Arabic and Hebrew, it relates to *Rekhem/Reham*, meaning "womb." The comparison is striking: the womb is where life begins, a place of nourishment, growth, and protection, all given selflessly. The womb symbolizes nature's inherent compassion—always in a mode of giving, expecting nothing in return.

This idea of selfless giving permeates creation. The sun shares its energy, enabling life through photosynthesis. Water rises from oceans, condenses, and falls as rain to sustain the Earth. Even within our bodies, every cell works in harmony to support the whole. The brain, for instance, consumes up to 25% of the body's energy, a testament to how resources are distributed based on need, not want. Compassion, at its core, fills gaps of inequality, ensuring balance and wholeness. The universe thrives on compassion and expects its creations to tread with caution.

The word "cautiously," its Arabic equivalent *Taqwa*, often translated as "caution" or "self-discipline," embodies the idea of prevention and restraint. Like a traveller walking along a path of thorny bushes would cautiously gather and secure their loose garments, mindful to prevent snagging and tearing on the sharp thorns. *Taqwa* gathers our desires, preventing destruction. When desires are unleashed unchecked, chaos ensues, and compassion—our healing force—is the first casualty.

This dialogue between God and the angels reveals the deeper laws of nature. It reminds us that humans, like cells within a body or denizens of the Earth, thrive only in balance. The choices made by our conscious self, the representative of our body's 100 trillion cells, figure out our health and well-being. Just as a society depends on wise governance, our inner world relies on the conscious self to act with wisdom and compassion.

Compassion is not merely a virtue—it is the thread that binds healing to harmony. The dialogue between God and the angels unveils a profound truth: the workings of the universe mirror the workings of the self. Just as the sun sustains life selflessly and the cells within us cooperate tirelessly, the balance of all creation depends on the choices made by its parts. This invites us to embrace a deeper understanding of the philosophical concept: as in the macrocosm, so in the microcosm.

The human body, with its trillions of cells, is a microcosm of the universe. The conscious self, much like a wise leader in a society, bears the responsibility of guiding this intricate system toward balance and well-being. By embodying compassion, we align with the fundamental laws of the cosmos, restoring the state of Ease inherent to our design.

INTRODUCTION

The prologue was just the beginning of my thoughts about how deeply connected our mind, body, and spirit really are. These are lessons I have learned through my own life. And like most lessons, they came when I was not looking for them, but through experiences, that shaped how I see the world today. Slow down and be mindful, for every moment reveals what you need to see.

Two parallel events in my life changed the way I looked at religion and health. One affects the mind, and the other affects the body, but both thrive on one's belief patterns, the belief being the die or groove of the mind through which all data, both internal and external, pass and come out in the shape of the die—the belief. The heat of the mind, after a threshold, is transferred to the body, which later becomes the ground for manifestation.

The root cause of all disease and illness—whether acute or chronic—is the mind. Some may argue that illness is because of a pathogen attack—viruses, bacteria, fungi etc., the microbes, but the fact is the human body, which is a conglomeration of 60-70 trillion cells, is already a bacterial soup.

The mitochondria—powerhouse of the cell, are bacteria in a symbiotic collaboration with other organelles of the cell I.e., in a give and take relationship. What remains now are bad microbes. Our immune system takes care of this with its evolutionary experience. Our mind which houses our beliefs, attitudes and habits is ultimately responsible for the breakdown of our defence system, as we shall see in the following pages.

As I reflect on these ideas, they bring me back to the stories of my own journey, a journey that begins with the story of my faith and the questions it raised.

Story No. 1

I was born into a Muslim family. All that is required to be a follower of any religion is one's birth into that religion, belief in a dogma, and carrying out certain rituals on a day-to-day basis. Like in other Abrahamic religions, there were angels, the devil, heaven, and hell all belonging to the invisible realm and belief required that one accept all these without questioning, but humans have a questioning mind. Against all odds, I grew up questioning, though they considered it a devil's act to question matters of religion.

What appeared to me as a dead end turned out to be a beacon of light—the Quran. I enrolled in a course wherein I learned the Quran word-for-word. My curiosity grew after finishing the Quran, leaving me with more questions. The Quran encouraged us to use our cognitive faculty, to question what seemed irrational but also required us to believe in the unseen. Many stories of the prophets had an element of supernatural phenomena. Then I began learning Classical Arabic, the language of the Quran, in an Academy named 'The Signet Academy'. A huge scroll-like painting was hanging at its entrance just above the door. The following unheard golden words were embroidered on a silk green satin cloth. More than the depth of the color, the words etched moved me.

muslims by birth Beware!

Lest you be confused I have addressed us with a small 'm';

Lest you take it for granted,

Islam is a way of life as revealed in Nature and is therefore everyone's birthright;

Lest you are mistaken Quran is an expression of all age-old truths and is a shared heritage of mankind;

Lest you are proud of your Heaven and others Hell, let there be a change of attitude with a pinch of humility for these states are strictly action-based; conditions do apply;

Lest you claim ownership over titles – Momin Muslim Mohsin Muttaqi,

Be aware that anyone who Submits to the Laws of Nature is a Muslim;

Anyone who vouches for Peace is a Momin;

Anyone who works to restore Balance is a Mohsin

Anyone who is in a Precautionary and Disciplinary mode is a Muttaqi;

Let go of wishful thinking;

The writing is clear on the horizon;

That if you are Momin you will be the most successful.

There was a paradigm shift in my thinking—no less monumental than the tectonic shift of plates. This transformation gave me the courage to question all the beliefs I had been running on autopilot. The next story is about the shattering of yet another belief, this time one deeply tied to health.

Story No. 2

During my college days in Keelakarai—a small coastal town just a few kilometers north of Rameswaram—I stayed in a hostel for the first time. It was there that I began experiencing a persistent pain at the junction of my oesophagus and stomach. I could feel acid being released even without food. Stress and excessive tea only worsened the situation, and homesickness compounded the problem. Being away from my family in Chennai, combined with the mediocre quality of hostel food and a lack of entertainment, only added to my woes. To watch a movie, we had to travel nearly 18 kilometers to Ramnad.

At the time, I relied on regular medicines to suppress acid production and soothe the symptoms with antacid gels. This routine continued until 2010 when my health took a turn. One day, I panicked after vomiting a blood-colored liquid. The reports confirmed a duodenal ulcer, and the doctors recommended an endoscopy. Hesitant but concerned, I agreed.

What followed changed my entire perspective on disease, doctors, and drugs. Something unexpected appeared in the reports that completely shifted my understanding of health. I share the full details of this ordeal in Chapter One.

This book reminds us of an important aspect of our body: it can heal itself. Therefore, it is a clarion call to humanity to return to its Nature, its origins—a state of Bliss, Joy, Harmony, Peace, or Ease not only with oneself but with every species that shares space with us on this planet Earth. Homo sapiens are the only species that have this evolutionary merit, wherein they are conscious of their consciousness. This aspect gives them the ability to create and empathize. They do this by seeing nature around them and then replicating their observations into technologies that have done more harm than good, on an individual level and a social level. Technology has given comfort and luxury, but at what cost? We used to walk miles, eat when hungry, and sleep after sunset. But with the invention of the Wheel and Light, everything went topsy-turvy. With wheels, we now have reserves of unused energy, and this gives rise to different lifestyle diseases. With light, we stay awake the whole night, consequently building up toxins that later manifest as diabetes, heart disease, tumors, ulcers, depression, and cancer.

This book is a transformational memoir wherein I hold a mirror to the readers so that they see where they are in their evolutionary journey of mind and body. The chapters that follow are not only stories of my struggle, but they have in them the grit you need to question your beliefs, attitudes, and habits. For this to happen the basic smallest requirement is to slow down and be aware of how you deal with your thoughts. Are they random or structured by your intention? Are they habitual or on demand? Likewise, you should be aware of your actions. Are they impulsive, instinctive, or well thought out for that situation? As we journey together, I would hold your hands and walk you through the various steps that not only removed symptoms from the periphery but healed me to the core.

This book is about a dynamic, self-sustaining system—our body—that works well when it aligns with nature by following the natural rhythms of our planet. The revolution of the Earth around the Sun causes the four seasons, the 29–30-day lunar cycle results from the Moon's revolution around the Earth, and the 24-hour day-night cycle is caused by the Earth's rotation on its axis. This idea is explicit in the Five Element theory discussed in Chapter Four, where each organ functions at its peak at specific times. If we do not align with these natural rhythms, there is a mismatch. We can neither calibrate nor standardize our bodies because consciousness is an abstract entity, enmeshed and entangled with each cell, making it impossible to quantify or arrive at a ballpark figure. A reminder that humans behave, while machines perform.

Disease to Ease is a journey from the fear of the unknown to the knowledge of how the mind and body work in tandem with the life force. Fear has many aspects to it. Apart from its physiological and psychological leanings, there is another aspect that the modern healthcare system fully exploits. The physiological response activates the flight-or-fight mechanism. This prepares the body to either confront or escape from a perceived threat. It does so by increasing adrenaline levels, raising the heartbeat to pump blood to the limbs, and quickening breaths. Stiffened muscles, dilated pupils for better vision, and sweating to cool the body during heightened activity are all part of this response.

The psychological aspect, on the other hand, motivates and influences behavior, creating a sense of unease, anxiety, or dread. It kindles the amygdala, the part of the brain associated with emotional processing, intensifying the emotional experience further. While this serves well as a survival mechanism in the short term, over the long run, it can have detrimental effects on mental health. In earlier times, when slavery was rampant, fear of punishment was the tool used to keep individuals as slaves. In modern times, fear is manufactured.

When a patient visits a doctor for some ailment, they are first recommended to undergo a battery of tests under the pretext of negating and ruling out any abnormalities. The problem begins when the results do not match the so-called standard parameters, as if the human body were a machine, forgetting that it is a dynamic system always approaching an equilibrium state. It would serve better if, instead of standardizing the parameters of BP, sugar, cholesterol level, creatinine level, etc.—the effects—we standardized human behaviors and attitudes—the causes.

Depending on the tests and their severity, the patient is awarded a life term imprisonment—diabetes, thyroid, heart disease, kidney failure, lung failure, liver failure, and, in worst cases, cancer. Depending on the vulnerability of the patient and the severity of the disease—sometimes based on the most difficult-to-pronounce name of the disease—the patient can die in 12 days to six months. Manufacturing fear first and then appearing as angels of healing! The wage of fear is death at every moment. Let us take the onus on us. We give in to fear first, further confirmed by our peers, relatives, friends, and then the most important group whom we trust completely, i.e., doctors, pharmacies, and labs. This is the story of overcoming fear.

From Disease to Ease is a journey—from a state of imbalance to that of balance. Health is the natural state of a body. The body always seeks an equilibrium state. Whenever there is an imbalance, disease occurs, and this not only affects the health of the body but also that of the mind. It becomes easy to understand the abstract functions of the mind when we study in correlation to the body. That is why they say, "heal the body, through your mind, and heal your mind, through your body".

I initially intended to divide this book into two parts: one focusing on Problems, where I would share my experiences with chronic and acute illnesses that my wife and I endured, discussing the various philosophies at work and our subsequent healing without medical intervention. The second part was meant to cover Prescriptions, the antidote for complete well-being that transcends cure and treatment to embrace holistic healing. However, as the book evolved, I realized that since our body is an evolutionary outcome, treating the book in parts would do injustice to the subject. Instead of dividing it into sections, I followed the trajectory of disease to ease through various experiences as they unfolded in my life, weaving a tapestry of a holistic approach to well-being. In effect, this book presents readers with a process distilled from a part of my life's journey.

The journey begins with my personal ordeal in Chapter 1. In Chapter 2, I recount how a thin, unassuming booklet became a source of strength and inspiration, instilling in me a deep longing for more. Chapter 3 introduces the wisdom and insights of a healer whose teachings profoundly changed me in ways I never imagined. Enamored by his approach, I attended a workshop, which I detail in Chapter 4.

In Chapter 5, we explore the Five Element Theory of Chinese medicine and its profound connection to health and harmony. Chapter 6 sheds light on the challenges women face before menopause and underscores the critical role of food as medicine in maintaining health.

The narrative shifts in Chapter 7 to a healer's relentless search for a complete cure for his daughters' mental struggles, uncovering approaches to heal fractured minds. Chapter 8 examines the vital distinction between treatment, cure, and healing, offering a deeper understanding of these concepts.

Chapter 9 emphasizes the importance of knowing and trusting one's body. This section highlights the awe-inspiring intelligence of the human body—how energy is distributed, how the immune system prioritizes survival by temporarily overriding the brain, and how balance is restored during regeneration.

In Chapter 10, we delve into the understanding that true healing must address all dimensions of the human being: Physical, Emotional, Mental, and Spiritual. This chapter encapsulates the journey toward a complete healing—from the periphery to the core.

Many books discuss disease and its prevention without drugs, but this one adds a crucial dimension to the root cause of illness—the degradation of social and moral values. As humans, we cannot afford to overlook these evolutionary tools. Lately, even conventional specialists have begun acknowledging the dangers of excessive drug use, invasive surgeries, and over-reliance on vaccinations. Yet, few have explored the deep connection between disease and the erosion of human values. Empathy, compassion, trust, discipline, humility, and—above all—selflessness are vital to our well-being.

So, let us empty our cups and begin the journey from *Disease to Ease*. No new knowledge can truly touch or transform us unless the mind is in a virgin state—a state of pure receptivity. May this journey broaden our minds and untie the knots that hinder our communication, understanding, and healing.

Discipline of Mind & Body is EASE.

An Indiscipline of Both – DISEASE.

CHAPTER 1

THE ORDEAL

The train was scheduled for early morning at 6:00, but we missed it.

A day before everyone in my family was happy. The occasion was my cousin's wedding in Mysore, and our entire clan was gathering there. However, my children's excitement was not about the wedding; it was about the journey.

I had booked tickets for the Shatabdi Express—a fully air-conditioned, superfast train of 2010 that zipped past smaller stations from Chennai, stopping only at three major stations, including Bangalore, before reaching its destination, Mysore.

My family— wife Salma, twin daughters Kulsum and Anjum, son Shuaib, and the youngest, Zainab— were eagerly waiting for me at home. It was 9:30 pm, and I was finishing the day's work, updating payment follow-ups with my partner, and wrapping things up for a 4-day trip that included sightseeing.

With quick steps, I headed to the parking lot, started my motorbike, and at once felt a sharp pain at the junction of my stomach and esophagus. Instinctively,

I rolled my head slightly downward, which eased the intensity of the pain. Somehow, I managed to reach home and rang the doorbell.

Salma opened the door and noticed something was off. "What happened, ji? You look pale and tired!" she asked, concerned.

"It's nothing, ji," I reassured her. "Just the same old acidic pain. I need to eat something to neutralize the excess acid."

She quickly served me my favorite meal: thick lentil gravy with aromatic spices, a puffed omelet, and rice. I ate gratefully, hoping the food would calm the storm in my stomach.

After dinner, I leaned back on the sofa, struggling to stay awake. I knew I could not fall asleep right away; lying down too soon risked a reflux—a condition where a burp reverses food out of the stomach. Depending on the acid content, this upward journey either burns the walls of the esophagus or temporarily soothes them with an alkaline effect. Fighting off sleep, I let my thoughts drift, preparing myself for the eventful days ahead.

My daughters were busy applying mehndi, laughter filling the air, when a sudden wave of nausea hit me. Startled by the retching sound, everyone turned toward me. Before I could understand what was happening, I vomited a blood-colored, watery liquid all over the sofa. The peach decorative pillow on my chest was now stained deep red.

Panic erupted. The sight of blood left everyone frozen for a moment. A storm of thoughts swarmed my mind—I feared this was the end, but I could barely speak.

"Kulsum! Call Mama!" cried Anjum, her voice trembling. Through half-closed eyes, I could see Kulsum fumbling with the receiver, her hands shaking as she dialed Ajaz, my brother-in-law, who lived nearby.

Before Ajaz could arrive, I vomited twice more in the same horrifying manner. I was told later that soon after, I became unconscious, having eliminated liquid stools darkened and soaked with blood.

It was 3 a.m. when Salma and Ajaz carried me into an auto and rushed me to the hospital. In the emergency room, a junior doctor on duty assessed my condition. He immediately administered an injection of Ranitidine.

"Doctor, why this injection?" Salma asked, her voice filled with worry.

"This is an H2-antagonist," the doctor replied mechanically, as if reciting from a textbook. "It reduces the acid secretion in the stomach, helping with ulcer pain, heartburn, or the healing of ulcers."

Then came the chilling warning: "It could be an ulcer. The bleeding might be from a wound in the intestine. If not treated in time, it can lead to cancer."

His words hung heavily in the air, sounding like a death knell. Salma's face paled as she gripped my hand tightly. A strange calmness washed over me, but deep inside, I knew this was just the beginning of a long and uncertain journey.

We had to cancel the trip to Mysore. My children were more than relieved to see me back from the hospital. I was frail and weak because of the dehydration but managed to wear a smile, especially for my youngest daughter, who was in tears seeing me in that condition.

The next day, everything seemed normal—except for the lingering blackish-red color of my stool, a probable sign of intermittent bleeding. Although the vomiting had stopped, every trip to the bathroom left me feeling weak, my legs trembling with exhaustion.

My co-brother-in-law suggested I consult a gastroenterologist, and within an hour, we found ourselves at a palatial multi-specialty hospital.

The specialist conducted a thorough examination and recommended an endoscopy. As he explained the procedure—how a thin, flexible tube with a camera would be guided down my throat—I felt my stomach churn, folding inward like the pleats of a saree. The very thought of it terrified me.

"I feel better now," I said, searching for an escape. "Maybe if the pain returns, we can consider the endoscopy."

But my wife, Salma, was resolute. "You're doing this now," she insisted. Reluctantly, I agreed.

I was led into a dimly lit room dominated by a wooden examination table and four glowing computer screens. The assistant gastroenterologist darted out a series of questions in a calm yet authoritative tone: "Were you on an empty stomach for at least six hours? Any allergies? Other health issues?"

"Lie down on your back and follow my instructions," he said reassuringly.

A nurse inserted a plastic mouthpiece—a snug fit designed to prevent me from closing my mouth. Through a central opening in the cap, the endoscope was carefully threaded in. As the tube reached the soft tissues of my throat, I felt an overwhelming urge to gag. The powdery lubricant coating the tube only worsened the sensation.

"Swallow when I tell you to," the doctor instructed. "It will help the tube glide down."

Each swallow felt like a battle, but I obeyed, fearing complications. I could hear the soft clicks of the camera snapping images inside me. The ordeal seemed endless, but finally, the tube was slowly retracted, and I was able to breathe freely again.

An hour later, the results were in. To my astonishment, nothing significant was detected. The commotion—the blood expelled through my orifices— was simply the result of a dried, crater-like depression in my duodenum. There was no active bleeding, no inflamed wound. The body, in its mysterious wisdom, had already begun to heal itself, much like a knife-cut on a finger mending over time.

Though my relief was immeasurable, it ignited a new curiosity in me. How had the body achieved such a feat? What mechanisms had worked behind the scenes? My search for answers began.

CHAPTER 2

THE JOURNEY BEGINS

As I was staring deeply into the images of my endoscopy's reports, trying to figure out what dried up the wound, I suddenly remembered my wife asking me this question a few days back before the incident: "Our body heals itself, it seems, can you believe this?" "Be careful about quacks," I snapped back. My wife was suffering from chronic gastric trouble. Her cousin had recommended her to an acupuncture healer. She visited the healer and was asked to follow these simple instructions: "Eat only when hungry. Chew well. Do not drink water just before and after meals. In case of emergencies, drink just to the level needed." "Was that all the healer prescribed?" I asked, surprised. She handed me a small booklet that had questions and answers about common health-related issues and the veracity of their healing methods.

With raised eyebrows and an air of skepticism, I took the book and randomly flipped through its pages. The flimsiness and the layout of the book made me do that. Otherwise, with a book, there is a ritual that I follow. First the Title, then the Back Page, followed by the Table of Contents and Introduction—all this with due respect and reverence.

Opening the first page of the book, I slowly straightened myself from the slouching posture. A particular line attracted my attention, and I completed the whole book in one sitting. It said:

"Disease is the result of a violation of natural laws!"

The moment our body experiences a violation, it warns. Warns each time, but we ignore. The basic function of the body and its smallest unit—the cell—is Digestion, to produce energy to live. Eating and excreting are the two functions of Digestion. Food has energy within. The metabolism that extracts this energy generates morbid matter or waste. The process of energy extraction has waste elimination built into it like two sides of a coin. These processes are separate activities; they are part of an organic whole. One without the other is inconceivable.

Therefore, a body is not a set of distinct activities like a machine but a self-sustaining dynamic system. This means digestion is not the function of the stomach alone; the whole body takes part in digestion.

- Digestion begins the moment food enters the mouth. Masticated food passes through the food pipe and enters the stomach.

- The spleen absorbs food energy the moment chewing begins.

- Bile from the liver and gallbladder aids digestion.

- The semi-solid paste is further broken down in the small intestine where the energy is absorbed, and the rest is sent to the large intestine.

- The large intestine removes energy from the undigested food and then solidifies it into feces before sending it out through the rectum. .

- The energy absorbed by the spleen and the small intestine is taken up by the red blood cells contained in the blood, transported to the heart, and from there circulated throughout the body.

- Kidneys recycle and absorb energy from the liquid waste. The leftover is expelled through the urinary bladder.

Thus, the entire body is involved in the digestion process, like an orchestra performing a symphony in perfect coordination, appreciated only as a holistic phenomenon but never in parts.

"Salma, can we meet this doctor for a second opinion on my endoscopy reports?" I asked, this time with due respect and reverence. The sincerity of the message and the wisdom in it were overwhelming filled with insights and curiosity.

The clinic was in Broadway near Parry's Corner, an area close to the harbor. As I negotiated through the traffic, I wondered how narrow this Broadway was.

Probably during its christening, this was the broadest roadway. With great difficulty, I managed to get a parking space and walked down a narrow lane. There was a billboard with a Yin-Yang symbol and the words *"AcuHome"* written in red. Beneath it was the tagline: *"Natural Healing Methods for a World without Drugs."*

There was a lot of commotion inside the hall. It was packed. An intro session had just concluded on their healing methods, and to my luck, I had all the senior healers and some who could converse in English as well. I waited outside, and there was a serene brightness on their faces. It appeared as if the entire atmosphere was charged. A few moments later, I was guided into the visitors' lounge. After a few minutes of waiting, I went to the healer's cubicle.

I wished him a hello and bent forward to hand over the reports. He just signaled with his palm not to. "What problem do you have?" he asked. "Everything is in the report," I reiterated. "These reports do not give a measure of the energy fluctuations that take place inside the body; they just identify the chemical changes that follow these energy fluctuations. That is all ok. Just tell me your problem." I narrated to him the entire ordeal, sequence by sequence, until I came to the endoscopy part. "When the vomits and motions ended, you were cured already. You should not have gone for the endoscopy because your wound was healed by the body. Without seeing the endoscopy, I can assure you that the reports would have been a big relief to you." I silently nodded.

"Doctors are men who prescribe medicines of which they know little, to cure Diseases of which they know less, in Human Beings of whom they know nothing"

- Voltaire

CHAPTER 3

HEALER, NOT A DOCTOR

The questions lingering in my mind needed answers, and I was determined to find them. This quest required me to question my beliefs, experience the opposite of what I had believed so far, and be open to ideas, concepts, and points of view from other systems of healing. The journey from one belief to another was arduous. A change of belief is akin to a new birth. But the pain involved in coming out of a belief is like abandoning the child one has nourished painstakingly. Though the human mind works on the principle of seeking pleasure and avoiding pain, people often go to extremes to safeguard their beliefs—taking millions of lives or laying down their own. Without beliefs, influence and persuasion would not have been the top-selling genre of self-help books. Beliefs are unquestionable.

To my inquiries about the modern healthcare system, I wanted answers from authorities—those doctors who had turned hostile toward their own system. To my surprise, there were many. They openly claimed that the modern healthcare system is a corporate business.

Wanting to understand more about the healing, I visited the healer once again to learn the secrets of his diagnostic methods and his understanding of the human body.

His stature had a commanding presence, with a voice and built that reminded me of a workshop I attended on voice modulation a few years back. The trainer had insisted that deep breathing for 15 minutes daily, combined with a disciplined regime of stretches and contractions, builds confidence and creates an aura of authority. To me, this healer of a gentleman was the epitome of my guru's teachings.

He greeted me with a smile and signaled me to sit down. Just behind him on the wall was an open bookshelf. Only the spines of a few hundred neatly stacked books were visible on the open bookshelf. Being a voracious reader myself, I could not help but sneak a preview of his interests. The genres ranged from Mind to Body, Cells to Civilizations, Chinese Medicine to Western Anatomy, and Medication to Meditation. I had to stop my scan as he was waiting with his question. "What brings you here?"

I was about to reply, "Doctor..." when he stopped me with a faint smile that just twitched the edges of his lips and said, "Call me a healer!"

"Is there any difference between the two? Because both work towards the betterment of the patients."

He leaned forward, his eyes reflecting a deep understanding as he explained patiently, "We healers do not just look; we observe. Your behavior, habits, and thoughts guide us to your core being." He was mentally tracing pathways of energy in the air—a balance of diagnosis and healing.

"On the physical front, we look for the patient's uneasiness by examining him thoroughly, and that would include any visible symptoms on the surface of the body—color, smell, emotions, likes, dislikes, and listening to the tone of their voice. All these are mere manifestations of some underlying imbalance, and after a complete diagnosis using the Five Element Theory, we balance the energy by tonifying if it is weak, dispersing if it is stagnant, or by sedating if the energy is in excess." There was a crackling sound of the leather-covered cushion as he relaxed back in his chair.

As I was the last patient for the day and finding me interested in the subject, he continued without an air of sarcasm: Doctors who have completed their degrees and pursued further studies following Western methods have a protocol checklist for diagnosis and treatment. They adhere to the Western reductionist method devised by René Descartes, the famous French philosopher and mathematician (1596-1650), whose quote is well-known to this day: "I think, therefore I am." When discussing the mind and body, he stated that both are separate entities, independent of each other, and that for any eventuality, the body alone is responsible. This means the mind, with its mental processes, thoughts, and consciousness, has no role in affecting the body. The division of the mind and body/brain as two separate entities is dualism.

To explain it from a health perspective: life—the driving force, the vitality by virtue of which a person is alive is enmeshed through each organ, tissue, muscle, sinew, lesion, nerve, cell, and fascia throughout the body. The mind, its mouthpiece, like life, is also entangled in more sophisticated and subtle ways. That's why it does not show up as a reading in any test report, X-ray, or scanning machine. However, there is a difference between the mind and vital life or spirit; when you're in deep sleep, an unconscious state, or a coma, the mind appears to be off, but there is life—breathing and heartbeat—which is quite apparent. The mind has actually switched off its senses, thereby devoting its entire focus to rejuvenating the whole system. Without this representative (mind), an efficient integration of the bodily systems is impossible. The mind gives direction to life. When the mind disintegrates, life becomes purposeless inside the body and therefore escapes, leaving the body lifeless.

When you (the mind) are low because of sorrow or grief, your body posture changes. A relatively dull environment is created within, inevitably affecting the workings of the heart (circulation), liver (detoxification), stomach (digestion), and lymphatic vessels (immune system).

The allopathy world treats the body like a machine. The way they calibrate a machine, they calibrate the body too, standardizing and holding particular values to be the norm for all individuals, such as blood pressure, body temperature, glucose levels, fat levels, creatinine levels, etc., entirely forgetting the fact that humans also have a mind—a consciousness—a consortium of memory, experiences, emotions, and imagination. Everyone has a distinct set of normalcy. What is fear for one may be an adventure for another. What is frustration or anger for one may be a way of soul-searching for another. Moreover, these calibrations are arrived at by following the law of averages, and the sampling quantity is too trivial compared to the varied range of human uniqueness with its vast range of emotions.

The healer's words unsettled yet enlightened me, stirring a mix of skepticism and awe. I chose my next question with care, my voice tinged with the uncertainty of a long-held belief that was never challenged. "What is meant by the reductionist method, healer?" He continued with the same fervor, although the purpose for which I had come was yet to be addressed.

He said, "Reductionism means dividing an entity into many parts and then treating each part as an individual entity without any connection among its parts. alienated from the whole. This theory suits machines well, not bio-organisms. Humans are conscious beings. Consciousness is an abstract phenomenon and cannot be quantified or calibrated because what is fear for one is an adventure for another."

"The opposite of reductionism is the holistic method. In a human body, there are no clear demarcations dividing the organs. One does not know where the heart ends and the lungs begin or where the diaphragm starts. Each organ gradually dissolves into another organ so gracefully, like day merging into night and vice versa, or a season changing into another harmoniously."

I asked if there was any healing method in the world that followed a holistic form of treatment. The healer responded, "Why not? And you will find a common thread running through these philosophies: healing the individual as a whole—not just symptoms but the root cause—transcending the body and mind to the life force." He then began to elaborate on other healing methods rooted in cultural and traditional approaches.

Ayurveda: The doctrine of Ayurveda aims to keep structural and functional entities in a state of equilibrium, which signifies good health. Any imbalance due to internal and external factors causes disease, and restoring equilibrium through various techniques, procedures, regimes, diet, and medicine constitutes treatment. The philosophy of Ayurveda is based on the theory of *Pancha Bhootas* (the five-element theory), of which all objects and living bodies are composed.

Siddha: The Siddha system of medicine emphasizes that medical treatment is oriented not merely to the disease but also takes into account the patient, environment, age, habits, and physical condition. Siddha literature is in Tamil, and it is largely practiced in Tamil-speaking parts of India and abroad.

Unani: The Unani system of medicine is based on established knowledge and practices relating to the promotion of positive health and the prevention of diseases. Although the Unani system originated in Greece and passed through many countries, Arabs enriched it with their aptitude and experience, and the system was brought to India during the medieval period. The Unani system emphasizes the use of naturally occurring herbal medicines, though it also uses ingredients of animal and marine origin.

Homoeopathy: Homeopathy is a type of medicine that started in Germany. It's based on the idea that 'like cures like'. This means that homeopathic doctors give patients diluted doses of portents made from minerals, metal, plants or even animal extract that mimic symptoms of the illness being treated. This stimulates the body's natural healing process.

Yoga and Naturopathy: Yoga is a way of life that has the potential for improving social and personal behavior, enhancing physical health by encouraging better circulation of oxygenated blood in the body, restraining sense organs, and thereby inducing tranquility and serenity of mind. Naturopathy is also a way of life, involving drugless treatment of diseases. The system is based on the ancient practice of applying simple laws of nature. Advocates of naturopathy focus on eating and living habits, the adoption of purification measures, and the use of hydrotherapy, baths, massage, etc.

In fact, **Traditional Chinese medicine** is also holistic in its approach. Remember we discussed life—the vital spirit enmeshed... Well, the Chinese call it *Qi* (pronounced chi). The primordial energy of the universe is *Tao*.

When a body is ill or diseased, there are different treatments to cure the illness. The word *curare* in Latin and Old French originally meant to take care of. Later, in Middle English, the sense of medical care was born. Curing means eliminating all evidence of disease, while healing means becoming whole. As you can see, the word *cure* refers to the disappearance of symptoms, while healing happens on a deeper level. There is an understanding that healing is a balancing act and an ongoing process.

One can cure chronic illnesses like digestion problems related to acidity, reflux, and heartburn by popping pills, but healing is possible only when one manages the person's eating habits, stress, worry, tension, and anxiety. In curing, there is the eradication of physical symptoms only, whether inside or outside the body.

Treatments are various methods used when there is no absolute cure, e.g., medicines that one takes for life, surgeries like open-heart or bypass surgery—where the chances of getting another block still looms large—or therapies used for paralytic attacks or psychological disorders, though the risk of recurrence stays.

Healing is not only the removal of physical symptoms but also the strengthening of the mind and spirit such that the quality of life improves. Healing is the restoration of health from an imbalanced, diseased, damaged, and un-vitalized organism, and it involves a human touch with compassion and empathy. Healing is holistic, tracing the imbalance of the body to its roots rather than merely treating symptoms."

In a subtle way, this healer explained to me with such strong conviction that the human body, being a part of nature, follows the same patterns and is also subjected to similar laws as that of nature. The way a forest recovers after a forest fire, our body too has the capacity to recover from any imbalances caused by a pathogen attack or toxic accumulation. The electron microscope and Magnetic Resonance Mapping might have reached the most intricate parts of the human body, yet the workings of the body are dynamic and cannot be standardized to suit our latest inventions and technologies.

It was already getting dark, and the healer offered me a ride to the nearest metro. My curiosity was unsatiated. "Healer! I want to know more about this subject. Can you share your knowledge and wisdom so that my family, friends, neighbors, colleagues, and relatives reap the benefits of holistic healing?" I asked.

"Why not? Attend a five-day workshop called *The Healer Within*," he replied.

I was excited and shared the conversation with my family at the dinner table. That was the last day our family members heard the word "Doctor." It was "Healer" from then on.

"The Healer Within" — something was mysterious about the title. So many questions were hovering around. Can the body really heal and take care of itself? If there is a Healer within, then where does it reside? If the body can heal itself, then why do doctors prescribe medicine, undertake tests, and recommend surgeries? What then about the latest research and advancements in medicine and medical equipment? With all these questions in mind, I was wondering, "Hope this is not another quackery or spiritual/energy healing." But somehow, I wanted to know what this was all about. The moment had come...

"When any part of your being is diseased or out of balance, gently bring it back into your Radar of Awareness, Healing begins..."

CHAPTER 4

THE HEALER WITHIN

Curiosity has a way of pulling you forward, and for me, it was now pulling me to the workshop. The promise of discovering The Healer Within felt like a journey worth taking.

The Healer Within. What a title! This was the moment I had been waiting for. So many questions hovered around, seeking answers. Can the body really heal and take care of itself? Is there truly a healer within, or is it just a poetic expression? The questions were simple, but their implications were profound, as they would eventually lead me to discover some of the most important existential truths about our creator, creation, and my role in it.

If the body can heal itself, then why do doctors prescribe medicine, ask us to take tests, and recommend surgeries? What about the latest research and advancements in medicine and medical equipment? And most importantly, vaccinations! With all these questions in mind, I yearned to clear my doubts during the workshop *The Healer Within*, hoping it was not just another form of quackery or spiritual healing.

On one hand, there are doctors, huge hospitals, the latest equipment, and diagnostic procedures that delve deep into the recesses of organs; on the other hand, we have these healers and whistle-blowers protesting, holding meetings at important junctions against the doctor-corporate hospital-pharma nexus, highlighting how people in third-world countries, living in low-income groups, are treated as guinea pigs for testing drugs before introducing them into the global market. An automated announcement jolted me from the dialectic debate playing out in my mind, just as the train hissed and screeched to a stop at Nehru Park station.

I gathered my thoughts and belongings and waited for the doors to slide open. It was 9:30 AM, and the workshop was to begin in another 30 minutes. The hotel was 500 meters away from the metro station. The doors opened, and I looked left and right for an escalator. Having spotted one on the left side, I walked a few steps, stepped onto the flat grooved surface, and waited for the loop to form a step. The moment it began forming steps, I climbed, despite its gradual ascent, to reach the venue faster.

Escalators have always fascinated me. It was 9:35 AM, but the mechanical engineer in me did not fail to take a mental note of this engineering marvel. What was even more marvelous was the body's engineering, from a single cell to a conglomerate of trillions. Even more awe-inspiring was the way the body transitions from a state of disease to ease. I recalled how my cold, cough, and fever had receded in three days without the help of drugs.

Reaching the exit, I slowed down my steps on seeing Abu Sarovar Portico, just two blocks away on the same side as the station.

The moment I entered the precincts of the hotel, there was a shift from the hustle and bustle of city traffic to a serene, silent environment. It was a different world inside. A lawn was hemispherically laid out with Kurian grass. On either side of the lawn were the exit and entrance gates. The periphery of the hemisphere was dotted with medium-sized trees. Opposite the lawn stood the portico, and on either side of the portico were two long 500-meter pathways that joined at the other end, giving the whole plot a rectangular shape. Cars and bikes were parked along those stretches on either side of the building.

At the entrance, a gentleman wearing a magnetic smile and an attire resembling that of the Maharaja mascot of Air India—royalty combined with humility— welcomed me inside. The heightened ceiling gave depth and serenity to the ambiance. The hotel's interior helped me regain my normal rhythm of heartbeat. I was on time.

It was 18°C inside the hall, and there were hardly any chairs left. A volunteer signaled me from the last row. The knock of my leather soles intermittently broke the silence as I walked to the chair. The gentleman who had coaxed me to attend the workshop was standing on the other side of the wall; he acknowledged my smile.

"Good morning, everybody!" greeted the speaker.

"Today, we have with us Dr. Raghuman—a revolutionary, our Guru, our Aasaan (a word of reverence in Tamil)—who has conducted extensive research and studies on Five Element Chinese Acupuncture. He later started the now-popular Indian Classical Acupuncture in Tamil Nadu. After completing his medical degree from a medical college in Chennai and a doctorate in medicine, he found himself dissatisfied with the current modern healthcare methodologies practiced in the name of treatment. He went on to challenge the concerned boards, including the All India Institute of Medical Sciences (AIIMS), criticizing their diagnostic methods and subsequent treatments. Today, he will brief us for a few minutes before we begin our workshop." Saying this, the speaker handed over the microphone to the doctor.

"Let peace prevail among us all, within and without," the doctor's voice resonated through the hall. I felt a stir within me—a mix of skepticism and curiosity that nudged me to listen more intently.

The doctor has thousands of followers across the state, Sri Lanka, and Malaysia. Every morning at his residence, starting from 5:30 AM, a long, meandering queue stretches from the main road to his bungalow, which is a few meters inside. The spectrum of his patients range from the common person to state

"Your behavior outside is copied by your cells inside. Be selfless for disease free life" ministers. With this aura around him, it was no wonder the entire audience was focused, not wanting to miss a single word spoken by him.

He continued, "I graduated from medical college in 1978 and was glad that the Almighty had chosen us doctors as saviors. I grieved at the fact that, how in the olden days slaves were given food only to the extent they could just survive and work. Nowadays, people are given information and knowledge about well being only to the extent that they can find their way to hospitals and serve their masters lifelong. The modern healthcare system was practicing tenets that were totally in contradiction to the Hippocratic Oath, which every doctor undertakes before being awarded a degree. His words echoed my own journey, from complacency with the modern healthcare system to a growing dissatisfaction with its limitations.

Let me reproduce part of the Hippocratic Oath from my memory:

I will prescribe regimens for the good of my patients, according to my judgment and ability, and never harm anyone. To please no one will I prescribe a deadly drug, nor give advice which may cause his death. Nor will I give a woman a pessary to procure an abortion. But I will preserve the purity of my life and my art.

Though the Hippocratic Oath, as seen through the prism of changing times, swearing to ancient Greek gods seems a little redundant in this multiethnic, multicultural, and pluralistic world, the fact remains that the oath embodies principles of beneficence, gratitude, confidentiality, and humility. These values are completely lacking in today's modern healthcare system. It functions as a corporate entity and therefore must generate profits. Patients become customers for a lifetime, which means they cannot be healed completely but must be checked regularly, much like the way a car is serviced, and after a sufficient run, undergoes a major overhauling.

To understand the way modern medicine works, we just need to consider its aftereffects. A sign of wellness is hunger, but with our drugs, the patient is left weaker and tired. If you have a problem with your eyes—say, you have short sight—what should happen after you consult a physician?"

"Sir! Normally, we should not have the problem after getting treated," shouted an enthusiastic youth from the fourth row.

"But does it happen that way?" asked the doctor, continuing.

"Normally, we prescribe glasses with lenses for short-sight, and each time you come for a check-up, the power increases, whereas healing requires that normal vision be restored. Well, the same is the case for any type of disease treated by Western methods, be it diabetes, blood pressure, heart disease—the list is endless. What is required is complete healing. Of all the healing systems that I can think of, I found the Five Element Chinese Healing system heals a person completely and suggests ways and means to live a long, healthy life. For this to happen, you need to understand the way your body works in tandem with nature's seasonal cycles. In the next few moments, you all will be learning how your body heals itself. I wish you all good luck!"

As he was praising his philosophy of healing, I couldn't help recalling my own futile treatments. His conviction made me wonder if this was the answer I had been looking for.

*It is not the germs we need to worry about.
It is our inner terrain."*

– Louis Pasteur

CHAPTER 5

THE PATHOLOGIST-TURNED-HEALER

As the second person took the stage, a flicker of recognition crossed my mind. I had seen him before. Our brain has this habit of recognizing patterns. It latches onto the nearest available pattern to give us a sense of safety and conserve energy—a survival skill and an evolutionary prerogative—because the brain consumes almost 20% of the total energy metabolized by the body from the air, water, and food we take in. Sometimes, the brain concludes that the person you are looking at resembles someone else, and sometimes it accurately identifies the actual person from memory with the right context.

Yes, it was him. He was one of the healers who had recently addressed a crowd that had completed a one-year diploma course in Indian Classical Acupuncture. I remembered him from the day before, when I had been to the Acuhome at Broadway for a second opinion. His badge read Amar beneath the bold inscription: "A World Without Drugs."

Dressed in simple attire, Amar exuded a quiet confidence that was both calming and commanding.

His presence was like a balm, soothing the restless energy of the eager attendees. His voice had a gentle yet firm timbre, resonating with the kind of wisdom that comes from deep experience.

"Before starting today's lecture, I would like to clarify a few things," Amar began in a tone that commanded attention. His words were simple yet profound, spoken in a mix of Tamil and English, ensuring everyone in the room could understand. "This five-day workshop is just the beginning. It's not about becoming a certified healer; it's about understanding your body, how it works, and how it heals. These techniques are for you and your family. If you wish to become a healer, there's a longer journey ahead."

As he spoke, I could sense a shift in the room. People leaned in, hanging on to his every word. He was not just imparting knowledge; he was awakening a sense of responsibility in us toward our own health.

Amar then delved into a personal story that had caused a paradigm shift in his thinking. "A fetus changed my life," he revealed, his voice tinged with a mix of sadness and revelation. He recounted his time in the paramedical field, where a heartbreaking incident at a hospital had unfolded. A young, childless couple had come in for treatment, and during the course, the wife developed complications. The doctor had recommended an urgent surgery to remove what was believed to be a tumor in her uterus. The surgery was performed, and the woman's life was saved. Amar's friend, who assisted in the operation, shared with him the details of the procedure. Curious, Amar went to the operation theatre to see the removed tissue. What he discovered there shook him to his core.

I remember the chill that ran down my spine as Amar described the aftermath of the surgery. In the dustbin, attached to the removed uterus, was not a tumor but a sixty-day-old fetus. The realization that a life had been mistakenly terminated was not only shocking but profoundly disturbing. Amar's voice broke slightly as he recounted how the doctor, upon realizing the mistake, had quickly masked his humanity with a cold professional facade.

"Let not anyone know about this," the doctor had warned, reducing a profound ethical dilemma to a mere occupational hazard. Amar's revelation was a stark illumination of the flaws and ethical challenges within the medical system.

I sat there, stunned. His story was a piercing critique of the medical system's fallibility and the ethical dilemmas it often presented. "Who is determining a child's life?" he questioned. "The doctor, the scan reports, or the entire medical system?"

He did not stop there. Amar Sir spoke of how, daily, normal people were turned into patients for the most ordinary of symptoms — a headache, a fever, a spell of dizziness — subjected to a barrage of tests and procedures.

This was the moment that set the stage for everything that was to follow in the workshop. I was captivated, my mind racing with questions and a newfound understanding of the delicate balance between medicine and healing. This was just the beginning of a journey into the profound depths of what it means to heal and be healed.

The incident with the uterus was far from an isolated case in the complex world of modern healthcare. Every day, it seemed, the medical system transformed ordinary people into patients. Common symptoms like headaches, fever, or dizziness – mere signals from our body announcing its detoxification efforts – were often escalated into causes for alarm.

I remember pondering the irony of blood tests. Veins, those carriers of impure blood to the kidneys for purification, were the very source of these tests. Drawing blood from veins to detect sugar or creatinine levels seemed to me equivalent to judging a house's habitability by inspecting its drainage pipes. It struck me as fundamentally flawed, yet this was the standard practice—a practice that rarely faced the scrutiny it deserved.

The medical benchmarks, those figures like 120/80 mm Hg for blood pressure, were not biological constants but averages derived from large population studies. They were mere correlations, not causes, and certainly not reflective of individual biological diversity. It was a one-size-fits-all approach in a field where individual differences were paramount.

The internet was rife with debates and discussions about these standards—many suggesting that blood pressure cuff measurements were outdated, advocating for more personalized techniques considering organ perfusion and cardiac function. Yet, the stronghold of clinical conservatism, insurance protocols, and pharmaceutical interests often silenced these progressive voices.

Professor Alfred North Whitehead's words echoed in my mind, "It requires an unusual mind to question the obvious." It seemed to me that, in our blind trust in the established medical system, we often overlooked the simplest questions, the most obvious flaws.

This reminded me of an incident with a friend. He was absorbed in a phone call on the terrace, oblivious to the iron pipes strewn around. In a moment of distraction, he tripped, and in a desperate attempt to balance, he twisted his ankle, which got caught between the rods. The X-ray confirmed a fracture, and there we were in the orthopedic surgeon's office.

The surgeon, a man of pragmatic brevity, explained the procedure. "I think you are aware of the process," he began, his eyes shifting from the X-ray in his hand. "It's straightforward. We drill holes at the ends of the bone to secure a metal rod alongside the fracture. This prevents bending and aids faster bone formation."

As I listened, it struck me how, even in our most vulnerable moments, we are often at the mercy of a system that views our bodies more as machines to be fixed than as complex, self-regulating organisms capable of remarkable healing. It was a system driven by protocol and prescription, often overlooking the body's innate wisdom and capacity for self-repair.

My friend hesitated before asking the surgeon a question that had been lingering in his mind. "Doctor, what happens to the holes at the ends of the bone once the rod is removed after healing?"

The doctor, with a reassuring nod, replied, "Not to worry. Through a process called calcification, those holes will fill up, and eventually, it will become whole bone again."

A thought crossed my mind, a question that seemed so obvious yet remained unasked: Why couldn't the natural process of calcification mend the fracture without surgical intervention? My friend, perhaps intimidated by the clinical setting, didn't voice this question. I recalled a similar situation with my mother, who had suffered a wrist fracture. Instead of opting for surgery, I had taken her to a naturopath. He carefully aligned the bones, securing them with a firm bandage to minimize movement. Three weeks later, the fracture had healed entirely – no surgery, no medication. It was a testament to the body's remarkable ability to heal itself.

Healing, I mused, is a noble profession, yet often it strays from its virtuous path. The medical field, heralded as a sanctuary of saviors, is mired in unsettling practices – from the commercialization of medical education to the corporatization of healthcare. It operates in a realm dominated by fear, from the anxious moments of pregnancy to the finality of the deathbed. The endless array of tests and interventions, all under the guise of prevention, leaves little room for choice or trust in the body's natural resilience.

I remembered another incident from a few years ago when the outbreak of Swine Flu had created a wave of panic. The widespread advisory to wear masks as a shield against the airborne virus had led to a frenzy of mask-buying. Yet, when I delved into the specifics, the absurdity became apparent. The size of the virus, minuscule at 0.004 to 0.1 microns, rendered the masks, with their 1-millimeter fabric gaps, ineffective. The virus could easily traverse these spaces, making the masks more a symbol of fear than an effective barrier.

This reflection brought me to a realization: what we truly need is a healing system rooted in empathy and understanding, not commercial gain. A system holistic in approach, acknowledging the body's innate wisdom and ability to heal. We need a transition from a state of chaos and fear—this widespread Dis-Ease— back to a natural state of Ease. It is time for a new kind of exodus, led not by traditional doctors bound in a corrupted nexus of pharmaceuticals and hospitals, but by healers who genuinely understand and honor the body's natural healing journey.

As Healer Amar delved deeper into the intricacies of Chinese healing methods, he illuminated a stark contrast to Western medicine. "Unlike Western treatments that often focus on symptoms," he explained, "Chinese healing addresses the patient holistically, encompassing body, mind, and spirit."

Intrigued by his explanation, I found myself pondering the often-misunderstood distinction between mind and spirit. With a mixture of curiosity and hesitation, I raised my hand. "Sir, could you clarify the difference between mind and spirit? It sounds abstract," I asked. My voice barely rose above the murmur of the room, and I noticed Mr. Amar straining to locate the source of the question. A volunteer quickly handed me a microphone, and I repeated my query, this time with a heightened sense of self-awareness.

Healer Amar paused thoughtfully before responding. "Consider this," he began, "when you write, the physical action involves your fingers—that's your body at work. The thoughts that guide what you write, that is your mind in action. But beyond these, there is a deeper dimension. The profound satisfaction, the fulfillment you feel deep within after you've expressed your thoughts, that resonates with your spirit."

His answer, simple yet profound, resonated with the audience. It was a moment of clarity, distilling the often-complex concept of holistic healing into an analogy that was both relatable and insightful. In those few words, Healer Amar bridged the gap between the tangible and intangible aspects of our being, shedding light on the essence of holistic health.

The Five Elements Theory

The room was quiet, the audience fully engaged by the clarity of Amar's explanation. As his words lingered, he transitioned to the next part of his lecture, linking ideas about nature, existence, and healing.

Amar started by sharing a story, transporting us to a time when humans were deeply attuned to the rhythms of nature. "Our ancestors," he explained, "were master observers. They recognized patterns in the natural world – the cycle of seasons, the lunar phases, and the daily turn of the Earth itself. From the grand orbits of galaxies to the microscopic play of atoms, and even the blood flowing through our veins, everything moved in harmony. This profound connection between the cosmos and the pulse of life on Earth led to the birth of the Five Element Theory."

I was touched deeply by this information. Every cell was longing to know more. I immediately realized that even our DNA, which contains our genetic imprint, is also a spherical helix. Observation is the key to understanding the underlying patterns of the Universe.

Amar delved deeper, linking the mysteries of the universe to human existence through three pillars of Chinese philosophy: the life force of Chi, the balance of Yin and Yang, and the foundational Five Elements. "These principles," he said, "are not just philosophical musings but practical tools that mirror the intricate play between the vastness of the cosmos and the intimate world within us."

"There is an all-pervading energy permeating all life forms, both visible and invisible. Even the forms without life, like rocks, mountains, and rivers—home to various life forms—have the same elements, compounds, and molecules that make up their affluent brothers. Dao, life force, Spirit—names in different languages, all mean the same and are the underlying causeless cause or the primal force that then divides into two: the Ying and the Yang. Their reactions give rise to Heaven and Earth, Day and Night, cold and hot; each pair represents a yin/yang relationship. This division in the unity of things, as represented by the pervading energy, is essential to discern and compare.

"Later, the Yin and Yang are further divided into the Five Elements, and the whole universe can be mapped with these elements.

"The Five Elements cycle is the simplest of concepts that lie at the heart of Chinese Healing. These elements, viz., Wood, Fire, Earth, Metal, and Water, actually represent the day-to-day observations of happenings in nature and within our own selves. Leading a life that is in harmony with the nature outside and nature within is the Chinese idea of spirituality."

The lady next to me, curiosity lighting her eyes, interrupted, "But Sir, how does this align with our traditional Siddha practices? If we are talking about being in harmony with nature outside, then shouldn't we be following our traditional system of Ayurveda or, to be more precise, Siddha?"

Amar smiled, ready to bridge ancient wisdom. "That's a good question," Amar acknowledged. "Though Siddha and Ayurveda also follow the *Pancha Boothaangal,* i.e., the Five Elements, the comprehensiveness with which Chinese philosophy maps the elements is rational and scientific, and it applies to other fields apart from health, viz. astronomy, Feng Shui, cuisine, music, and even governance during the olden days."

"All traditional healing models have based their treatments on the constitutional makeup of individuals because each one is unique," continued Amar. "This therefore means that the reason for high blood pressure in Jack is definitely different from that of Jill, and this difference depends on the physical, mental, and emotional makeup of each individual."

"As mentioned earlier, these laws are derived from nature by observing the changes elements undergo in a year with a corresponding alteration in the plant world. The birth of a bamboo shoot represents the Wood element or Spring season; its blooming into flowers represents the Fire element or Early Summer; the harvest or the period of fruition represents Earth or Late Summer; the falling of leaves during Autumn represents Metal; and the final drawing in of life energy of the tree with its bare branches during Winter, representing stillness and tremendous potential, is the Water element. It contains the seed for a new birth in Spring.

Wood symbolizes the early birth stage, beginning, and development of life as it unfolds according to the plan inherent, as in a seed. Fire symbolizes the period of maturity and luxurious growth, where life reaches its zenith, like the sun at noon. Everything is in light and full expression. Earth refers to the first decline from adulthood, as the light wanes from maximum intensity during noon. It symbolizes abundance, stability, and nourishment, as observed during harvest time. Metal symbolizes the setting of old age and is a period of tranquility or calmness, where energy continues to diminish. It is a time to let go, as the active stages of life are done, and one gets in touch with the quality of life. Water symbolizes death, where energy is now turned inward. It is a time to go into the depths and return to the source of life, to burst forth once again with rejuvenated energies and experiences."

"The Five Element cycle is a circle, where wood gives rise to fire, as in the case of a log serving as fuel to a fire. Fire produces earth in the form of ashes. Earth begets metal in her womb in the form of minerals and ores or mountains rising from the plains. Metal holds water, as in the rivers that run down a mountain or in the rocks of streams that hold water in place. Finally, water, the source of life, allows the trees to grow, thus creating wood again and completing the cycle. This is a creative cycle where one element is created out of another. It is also known as the Mother-Child cycle.

"There is another cycle called the Control cycle. In this cycle, wood controls earth in the way trees prevent hillsides from eroding; earth controls water as the banks keep a river in its course; water controls fire since it can put out a blaze; fire controls metal in that fire can melt metal; and metal controls wood in the way an axe can fell a tree.

"The Control cycle is important to check the energy build-up that could lead to imbalance. Imbalance can also occur when the energy is insufficient.

"Having observed the connection of the Five Elements with various aspects of nature, it's now time to relate these elements to the human body, as we too are extensions of nature." Alan Watts, the American Zen philosopher, once remarked, "Organized religions have us believe that human beings are a special creation; they have been endowed with powers to control nature; that all species are subjugated to them. The fact is, human beings are not dropped from heaven but are products of earth, the way leaves grow out of branches in a tree."

To make the ancient wisdom of the Five Elements resonate with our lives today, Amar suggested simple daily practices. "Observe the changing seasons, feel the elements within you, and you'll start to see how closely linked we are to the world around us," he advised.

How the Five Elements Theory Shapes Our Lives

The connection between the Five Elements and our lives became increasingly clear as Amar guided us further. With each element representing aspects of nature and patterns within us, the wisdom of the ancients began to take shape.

The wise of the ancient world applied these Five Elements to the human condition. Once we understand that we are a microcosm reflecting the same patterns as the macrocosm, each of the elements holds a meaning to our lives and provides a system of healing from imbalances. Reading the energy changes in a person would have remained an intellectual endeavor were it not for the evolution of practical ways to read these energies through the senses.

Wood signifies growth, creativity, and evolution. The green shoot of bamboo that reaches for sunlight, a single zygote evolving into a human, or bringing ideas into realities—in general, giving form to the formless— all signify the workings of the wood element. When balanced, we approach life with assertiveness and a clear vision, much like a bamboo navigating through the cracks of a sidewalk. But imbalance can manifest as frustration or anger, the way a plant struggles in inadequate light.

Since wood symbolizes growth and development, all we need to observe in a person is whether their life contains new births—creativity as found in nature. Is there a plan, a vision of where they are headed? Can they make the decisions that allow growth?

"Prolonged Irritation Manifests as Anger."

*"Prolonged Anger Manifests
As Gall Bladder Stones."*

*"Stones look good On Ornaments
Not In Organs."*

Since balance is the criterion, a healthy expression of the wood element in humans is assertiveness, like the expanding bamboo shoot that pushes up through a crack in the ground. When this activity goes to the extreme, or when growth does not occur in a person's life, the tension and frustration may be reflected in a voice that shouts and in emotions of anger—expressions identified as the wood element out of balance. The ideal balanced condition would be to express a range of emotions and not get stuck in one, like children who are angry one moment and forget and move on the next. On the other hand, if the wood element is deficient, one may not be able to assert themselves, may not have the creative energy to initiate changes, and hence be unable to grow. During spring, the color is green; the phrase "green with envy" indicates an awareness of this phenomenon. The odor is rancid, similar to a locker room in a gym.

Defined as the child of water in the creative cycle, it draws on the energies of water, light, and wind into a coherent stem. In other words, it emerges from a coherent whole to express itself as an individual form.

The second aspect of the wood element is individuation—forming boundaries, creating individual egos out of universal consciousness. We see in nature that a tree is firmly rooted to the earth at one end and reaches the sky at the other by turns and twists, bending and reshaping its trunk as conditions change around it.

This brings us to the third aspect of the wood element—firmness and flexibility. In the Control cycle, the sharpness of metal cuts through it, thereby limiting or directing its growth. Wood expresses itself in movement and direction, indicating its potential energy and ability to change.

As Amar delved deeper into the elemental influences, he shifted our focus to how these elements manifest in our interpersonal relationships and self-perception.

Interpersonal relationship ability to communicate, make connections, and develop true intimacy are all characteristics of the Fire element. The Fire element represents our capacity for warmth and connection. Picture it as the glow of a campfire drawing people together. Balanced, it nurtures love and joy; unbalanced, it can lead us to feel cold and distant, or alternatively, to seek happiness in ceaseless social activity without finding true contentment. Love comes as a deep spiritual experience of this element. Too much redness is an imbalance along with inappropriate laughter, excessive joy, or a lack in these qualities.

The odor is scorched, like the smell of a hot iron kept on clothes for too long. People who lack warmth, who cannot make a connection, who seem cold and distant, and lack the spark are all victims of Fire element's imbalance. Then there are those who are always laughing and socializing, who are never happy unless they party constantly, seeking joy, is also an indication of lacking a genuinely sustained Fire element on the inside.

The Earth element offers a foundation, like fertile soil allowing a seed to sprout and grow. It's about feeling secure and nurtured. An imbalance might show up as anxiety or over-caretaking, mirroring a field either barren or over-fertilized, neither of which supports sustainable growth. Earth energy is all about stability and a sense of being grounded to the human condition. Insecurity indicates that a person is struggling in this element. Late summer is the time of harvest. In assessing an individual's Earth, we may ask whether she feels nurtured, can nurture others, and can bring forth a harvest in her life.

A yellow color is seen along the side of the face when there is an imbalance. The sound of singing and the emotion of sympathy remind us of a mother caring for a child. An imbalance would be a person inclined to be a mother for everyone or who is constantly seeking sympathy or is lacking in sympathy. All these are imbalances in the element. The odor is sweet fragrance, and an interesting correlation is that people having uncontrolled diabetes (a disease of the pancreas, which is an organ associated with the Earth element) have a fruity smell of ketones on the breath and urine.

The elements represent the natural world and reflect our internal states, shaping the way we navigate life's challenges and transformations. This deeper connection reveals how profoundly we are tied to the cycles of nature.

Metal reflects our search for meaning and the value we place on ourselves, akin to finding precious minerals within the earth. An imbalance can lead to despair, as if we are mining in vain for a sense of worth, or conversely, hoarding material wealth as a substitute for deeper fulfillment. Metal is required for self-esteem and, in extreme cases, leads to despair and depression. When imbalanced, the color white, like the sheen of metal, may appear; a weeping voice, emotions of grief, and a rotten odor, similar to a decaying pumpkin, are evident. Though this metal has little to do with material possessions, people try to compensate for a deficiency by acquiring money and jewels, which are physical manifestations of this element.

People seeking gurus across the globe in jungles and mountains are often searching outside for what they are missing and can only find within.

Water stands for the depth of our reserves and the ability to rest and regenerate. Think of a tranquil lake reflecting the sky. Imbalance might appear as exhaustion or an inability to flow with life's changes, equivalent to a stagnant pond or a flood eroding the landscape. Water symbolizes a time of stillness and rest that allows for the building up of reserves. When the reservoirs are dry, there is no potential for life. A deficiency in this element may result in a severe depletion of energy. Water brings fluidity, freshness, and the ability to flow; a person lacking this element becomes rigid. A groaning sound in the voice or darkening under the eyes indicates an imbalance. The associated emotion is fear—fear of drowning or a fear of scarcity in the storehouse during winter. Appropriate fear is necessary for safety and survival, but unnecessary, constant risk-taking is also a sign of imbalance. The odor is putrid, like stagnant water, dampness, or the smell of urinals.

The interconnectedness of the Five Elements goes beyond emotions and behavior; it is deeply linked to our physical bodies. This connection between nature and our internal systems becomes clearer when observed at the organ and cellular level.

Expression of Five Elements in Organs and Cellular Level

Fats are associated with Wood since they are digested with the aid of the gallbladder and are processed by the liver.

Proteins, the spark of life, are related to the Fire element. The organs are the heart, small intestines, pericardium, and triple warmer.

Carbohydrates are considered to be the expression of Earth, as they provide the sweet taste, while the pancreas produces the insulin needed so that sugar is checked and certified for consumption by the cells. The stomach and spleen are the organs associated with the Earth element.

Both the minerals needed for healthy functioning and the oxygen required for respiration correspond to Metal. The organs are the lungs and large intestines.

Water comprises two-thirds of our bodies, carrying out irrigation and elimination work through the kidneys and urinary bladder.

Patterns repeat in nature. As the saying goes, "ocean in a drop." Amar was visibly excited when delivering this sentence: "in the microcosm is the macrocosm."

The interconnectedness of the Five Elements and their expression in the body naturally leads us to another profound concept: the holographic nature of our being. This principle reveals how every part of our body is a reflection of the whole, making it a remarkable system of interconnected intelligence.

Our Body – A Hologram

The holographic principle states that all the information contained within a region of space can be figured out by the information on the surface holding it.

The beauty of our body lies in its holographic nature. We all know that our entire body can be mapped on our palms, soles, ears, face, or even in the eyes and tongue.

This is possible because our organs, though fixed in a particular location inside, have their functions represented all over the body—both on the exterior and interior—not just in that specific place. Representatives of all the organs are spread throughout the body.

To give you an example: Neurons are not only found in the brain; they are also found in the heart, the gut lining, the skin, the spinal cord—in fact, everywhere throughout the body. Similarly, it is not only the heart that pumps blood; the arterial walls, including the capillaries and blood vessels carrying the blood, have an endothelial lining that performs the pumping function too.

What is the impact of all this information? It's this: disease or illness is not localized. The whole body is ready to challenge it without any outside intervention. As a faithful representative of the approximately 100 trillion cells, what the body expects of us is to support it during its balancing act.

How? By aligning our will with the will of the body. This alignment comes from understanding its workings. It can only happen when we are thoroughly familiar with our inner terrain—our energy distribution via meridians to various organs, our immune system, our intra-body communication, our microbial allies, and what diet could empower our body.

As we think about how everything in our bodies is connected, it's clear that our health relies on a delicate balance. Each element and organ plays a part in keeping us well. But what happens when this balance is disturbed? When things go wrong, and we feel out of sync? This question leads us to a moment that demonstrates how deeply we can feel the effects when our body's natural balance is disturbed. It's in these challenging times that the principles of healing aren't just ideas; they become real and essential, guiding us back to wellness.

*"Fire in you is for Digestion & Passion not
for Jealousy & Anger;*

*For the Former kindles Creativity and the
latter leaves Ashes."*

CHAPTER 6

A PAUSE THAT LINGERED

Little did I know that I would soon confront these ideas on a deeply personal level. I was in a deep sleep in the new independent house we had rented a few days back when I heard a sobbing sound. It was around four in the morning, and with great difficulty, I opened my eyes to see my spouse standing in front of the mirror. She was looking frail, weak, and had a bloated stomach—an image she could not digest.

I tried to comfort her with all the persuasive techniques and healing knowledge I could muster at that early hour. Our son's wedding was three months away, and she had lost 12 kg.

A few months ago, she had been normal managing the boutique, designing exotic bridal wear, taking part in and sponsoring shows involving celebrities and upcoming models, dancing and playing with grandchildren, and turning out mouthwatering delicacies from our kitchen. To sum it up, she was living a life that defied her age, and her relatives saw her as an ideal to be followed.

There was tremendous pressure from my in-laws to scan her body and check for any tumors. As a healer, I knew what would follow would be results from a diagnostic lab. But I did not want to impose my views on my spouse.

"Take the call," I said.

"Nothing, ji, nothing is going to happen to me. I have not taken a single drug, I have not suppressed a cold, a fever, or a cough, except for the last delivery, which was a C-section—and I would not have accepted that too had I known what I know today," she said. "I am just crying over my state and appearance."

When the pressure was mounting, I said, "Consult with a doctor of your liking. But one thing is for sure, I would not go with you," to reiterate my confidence that the body can heal itself. However, her siblings wanted to take her to an Unani doctor.

Despite the pressure, my wife was firm. "Take me to your acupuncture healer," she said, her voice resolute. "I trust that method more than modern health care."

He employed a blend of Chinese traditional medicine diagnostics, which included pulse reading followed by needling at acupuncture points determined after a complete hearing of the patient's symptoms. This was complemented by a regimen of Siddha diet recommendations. His holistic methods resonated with her beliefs about conventional medicine, aligning with her own cautious stance.

Weeks passed, and while the symptoms eased slightly, it was not enough. The healer's methods were helping but not fast enough. It was then that desperation pushed me to consider other options. One morning, as I flipped through a health magazine, an ad caught my eye—Advanced Nutrition Course, Lincoln University, Malaysia, under Dr. Biswaroop Roy Choudhary. My mind raced. Could this be the missing piece we needed?

The program was set to start in a month, and I knew I could not waste time. I had previously learned under Dr. BRC in Bhopal, and his insights had changed my perspective on healing yet again. Now, more than ever, I needed those insights. I needed to find the missing piece of the puzzle.

Before diving into the details of the journey, allow me to take you on a little detour…

David vs. Goliath

The journey into alternative healing had already reshaped my understanding of health and the body's innate capacity to heal. Yet, as I ventured deeper into acupuncture practice, I found myself confronting a new set of challenges—both from the patients and within myself.

When I started my acupuncture practice, skepticism hung in the air like clouds during a storm. Patients arrived with furrowed brows and hesitant questions, doubting how a mere touch could start healing.

Their doubts were understandable; after all, the intricate philosophy of acupuncture was a mystery to many. Their questions were predictable: "How can you treat anything without medicine? How do you reduce a tumor without any diagnosis? And without frequent checks—blood pressure, sugar levels—how do you ensure health is maintained?" These doubts stemmed from gaps in knowledge and a lifetime of being taught that healing must always involve pills, diagnosis, and constant monitoring.

All that was needed to convince the patient was health recovery during the first sitting. My doubts were of a different nature because I had already passed through the first level of skepticism when I was suffering from chronic acidity, which ended up as an ulcer. There were still a few blind spots in my understanding of acupuncture, especially those pertaining to the food we eat and how intention alone had so much power to kickstart the energy flow through the meridians. This energy is the life force behind the movement of blood, hormones, enzymes, neurotransmitters, protein, and glucose molecules in our bodies.

To provide a rational explanation for acupuncture's healing effects, I began seeking more concrete evidence. I immersed myself in research, consulted experienced practitioners, and even experimented with various techniques to see what worked best. My goal was not just to heal but to empower my patients with understanding, so they could embrace this method with confidence.

When an ordinary man rises for a cause that benefits creation in its entirety, he becomes extraordinary. He overcomes his problems first and then goes on to help others. Nature starts revealing her secrets from her bosom when she knows for sure the secrets will be shared unconditionally without any commercial considerations. Such people work against the norms that are common: removing disparities and bridging the gap between the haves and have-nots. The masses initially avoid them but later, when they see results, they proclaim them as Saviors, Messiahs, Avatars, and whatnot.

To achieve the objectives mentioned above, in ancient scriptures, we find an individual standing up against the atrocities and exploitation rampant in their societies that are normally ignored by the masses. In spite of abuse, threats, and violence unleashed by the upholders of the existing system, this uprising gathers momentum. The individual establishes a new order of things among his followers, with clear-cut goals and a training program that has the double responsibility of erasing age-old beliefs implanted since aeons and making them live in accordance with the true knowledge that upholds the universal values of Justice, Equality, and Liberty, devoid of exploitation.

History repeats, and nature always works in patterns, and there is a never-failing consistency to them. Only then are we able to discover laws of Nature—from gravitational to buoyancy. This is the story of a person who is very much alive and very much Indian, Dr. Biswaroop Roy Chowdhury. He holds a doctorate in Diabetes and was mentored by Colin Campbell, the author of 'The China Study,' and the doctor who was instrumental in healing former US President Bill Clinton of his recurring blocks despite a few bypasses and open-heart surgery.

The journey of extraordinary individuals often starts with a singular realization—a deep understanding that compels them to challenge norms and empower others. Such was the case with Dr. Biswaroop Roy Chowdhury.

"Health is the natural state, and illness is a result of carelessness manifested as imbalance.

Taking medicine is an irresponsible act in these times. What is the solution if there is no cure? How do we avoid pain and discomfort?"

These thoughts became the impetus to kick-start a movement to empower the masses with the knowledge of how their bodies have the innate capability to heal themselves and to understand the difference between medical science and the medical industry. The latter, an exploitative tool, extends its talons into the food industry as well—first luring people with ready-made, processed, and preserved foods that are nutritionally deficient, and later casting a dragnet of tests and parameters required for "health," thereby creating a shadow of fear about what may go wrong if these parameters are not adhered to.

*"Illness is always due to errors
of diet & manners of living;*

*Germs are present solely as
scavengers of dead and waste tissues,
not the cause of Disease"*

– Antoine Bechamp

Dr. Chowdhury first introduced his DIP diet program, based on the concept of nourishing the body with uncooked food that has a molecular structure similar to digestive enzymes. These enzymes, ever ready to receive food when we are hungry, work seamlessly from saliva in the mouth to the digestive juices secreted in the stomach and small intestines.

With the help of a simple analogy that everyone could relate to, BRC made complex scientific concepts easy to comprehend and follow. The underlying idea behind the DIP diet was this:

Near a traffic signal in the Indian scenario, while everyone is waiting for the signal to turn green, a VIP car with a red-light cuts through the traffic and jumps the signal. But the disciplined, intelligent people (DIP) wait for the signal to turn from amber to green and then move on.

Similarly, the food we eat, as it enters the stomach, is supposed to wait for some time before it is absorbed into the blood. Fresh vegetables, legumes, wholesome grains, fruits, seeds, and nuts are disciplined and intelligent substances that wait for the signal—digestive enzymes in this case. They scan the food, and it is a sort of handshake allowing the food to drip into the blood and later on is broken into its constituents, gradually absorbed into the blood, and transported to various cells.

However, food that is grown with fertilizers, manufactured with preservatives, and processed does not wait in the stomach but rushes into the blood. There is no handshake with the digestive enzymes. They behave like the VIP vehicle that does not wait at the traffic signal. The blood sugar shoots up as the entire food is sugar-rich, stripped of all the essential nutrients like fibers, antioxidants, and enzymes that would otherwise aid in breakdown and slow the absorption. Since the absorption is immediate, it becomes difficult for the pancreas to cope with this sudden insurgency. The main function of the pancreas is to facilitate the entry of glucose (sugar) into the cells, and this it does by releasing insulin. Insulin gives step-motherly treatment to processed food for the following reasons:

- High glycemic index: Processed foods are often high in refined carbohydrates, which means a rapid spike in blood sugar levels as discussed above. This irregular insulin behavior.

- Low fiber content: Fiber, which helps in slowing down carbohydrate absorption, is low in processed foods making it more difficult for insulin to manage blood sugar levels.

- High sugar content: Processed foods contain added sugar. Why do processed foods add sugar? They do it to improve shelf-life as sugar acts as a preservative; to maintain structure and consistency in processed foods so that it doesn't appear stale and worn out; to enhance flavor; for cost-saving as sugar is the cheapest ingredient; for masking bitterness; and finally,

• sugar is a great binder holding other additives together.

- Unhealthy fat content causes inflammation, clogging of the receptors in the cells, excess acid in the blood—all these factors disrupt insulin behavior.

- Lack of nutrients: Our body is intelligent and doesn't waste its secretions on processed foods whose nutrient value is zero when compared to natural foods that are of high nutritional value.

On the other hand, natural foods are:

- Whole and unaltered

- Grown or raised in nature

- Not processed or altered

- Higher in nutrient and fiber content

- Lower in glycemic index (slower absorption into the blood)

- More satiating

- Supportive of healthy gut bacteria (microbiome)

Taking all these into consideration, BRC developed a diet program that included the goodness of natural food while not depriving people of their habit of consuming cooked food. The basic DIP diet is as follows, though variations exist depending on the individual's health.

- Avoid animal products, including including milk-based products like curd, buttermil, milk sweets etc.

- Eat fruits (10 x Body Weight) grams for breakfast.
- Lunch will comprise two plates:
  - Plate No. 1: Fresh vegetables (5 x Body Weight) grams, uncooked and unboiled.
  - Plate No. 2: Normal food, minus animal products.
- Dinner will be similar to lunch but must be completed before 7 p.m.

This type of diet regularizes blood sugar and blood pressure in 3–5 days. As more people started benefiting from his DIP diet, he introduced newer concepts of healing that incorporated the best of ancient holistic healing methods backed by the latest findings in molecular biology, nutrition science, and the role of good microbes in metabolism (microbiome). His methods were always supported by proofs, journals, and research papers accepted worldwide by scientists but not shared with the masses for commercial reasons.

Steadily, he structured his philosophy of healing into these few guiding principles:

- Fastest
- Safest
- Evidence-based
- The most economical
- No side effects
- Available to all

Philosophers are accused of ranting and bragging about their ideas, but BRC believes in action. To achieve the above, he employs:

- Food as Medicine
- Time as Medicine
- Light as Medicine
- Earth as Medicine
- Gravity as Medicine
- Movement as Medicine

True to Dr. BRC's intentions, all the above-mentioned tools are available as books for everyone to read on his website. I have dealt only with Food as Medicine to share the results of applying his philosophy.

Even as I write this, Dr. BRC has proposed launching 500 clinics across India, aiming to empower the masses by dispelling their fears and educating them on self-care.

Returning to our old story—it was pandemic time, and the classes were online. I started applying the principles even as I was pursuing the course in Advanced Nutrition. There was further weight loss, but the water retention that caused the bloating of the stomach persisted. I was in a demanding situation and on the verge of losing hope. Suddenly, it dawned on me that the water retention was due to a lack of energy needed to move the water to the kidneys from the small intestine—this was the area of retention. The energy was being used up by the stomach for digestion.

I recalled an entire subject during the workshop "The Healer Within" by Healer Amar, about how energy was distributed. (More of this in the chapter on Know your Body)

With caution, I approached my wife and asked, "Is it possible for you to be on a liquid diet for a day?"

"...Without salt," I added in a hesitatingly muffled voice.

I knew I was asking for too much, given her weight loss. But when I explained to her the science behind this, she agreed to it at once.

On the first day, she experienced diarrhea and vomiting. By the second day, she had regained her appetite and was sweating profusely. The bloated stomach was slowly deflating. The liquid diet demanded minimal energy for digestion, and since it was a salt-free diet, the kidneys were also cooperating. The extra energy at disposal was able to remove the excess retained water and significantly raise her energy levels.

By the third day, there were no mood swings, and her mind was brimming with positivity. I decided to taste her saltless diet, and tears welled up in my eyes at the amount of pain she was enduring to heal herself. Modern healthcare philosophy focuses on reducing pain and discomfort in the shortest time possible, often without concern for the side effects that can take their toll. However, she chose the longer route, one without side effects, and her decision yielded rich dividends.

Just as nature springs back to life after a silent, dormant winter, she too was bubbling with renewed vitality. With a stronger belief in the innate ability of the body to heal itself, she rose like a phoenix from the ashes, renewed and full of life.

CHAPTER 7

THE FRACTURED MIND: UNDERSTANDING THE BODY-MIND CONNECTION

The resilience of the human body is matched only by the complexities of the mind. Just as the body finds ways to heal itself, the mind often grapples with its own struggles, sometimes in ways that are harder to decipher. This became evident during a conversation about postpartum stress and its toll on mental health.

Postpartum stress, sleepless nights with a newborn, a short visit to Pune immediately after a long drive from Ooty to Chennai, followed by the excitement of her cousin's wedding, had noticeably affected the tone and texture of her voice. Every sentence ended with inflections and questions—that was not her normal self. She was the elder of the twin, the most responsible daughter in my friend Selvam's family. Normally authoritative, she had a commanding presence and could control sibling battles with just cold looks and stares.

That night at the dinner table, the decibels were higher than usual, and Selvam knew for sure she was experiencing a manic episode.

In manic episodes, the conscious self is in revelry of sorts. There are streams of consciousness, representing every single thought—either fantasies or past experiences lodged in the subconscious mind—trying to seek the light of day through the single conduit dashboard of awareness. The check valve, which typically allows only one thought to pass through after due social considerations, seems to malfunction and is effectively in a coma itself. This is likely due to the heavy load of gushing thoughts with unbridled energy seeking expression at once.

Sleep is the solution, but sleep becomes elusive as the individual struggles to resolve or discipline the thought flow. It is a night of lights for the mind—a paradox of mental illness.

Is there a way out?

Coming back to our story, the other twin, under the pretext of taking care of her sister, also spent sleepless nights and became a victim of twin syndrome. So, it was hell on fire! Selvam, who had in fact studied all those courses related to holistic healing with me, found his learnings and philosophies thrown for a six because this was an emergency, and the ways of holistic healing were more focused on prevention and precaution. It was then that I reminded him of the golden words of another allopath turned naturopath, "In case of emergencies use allopathic medicine, once the situation is under control, then get back to your natural state of holistic healing."

With great reluctance, he consulted a psychiatrist. The first thing these drugs did was,put them to sleep. By the third day, they were normal. After tapering the drugs with the help of a psychiatrist turned homeopath, he resorted to cognitive behavioral therapy (CBT).

The premise of CBT is that it is not what you think that affects the mind, but it is what you feel about your thinking that makes the difference. It helps reframe negative thought patterns and improve coping mechanisms, supporting mental health.

The gross part of the mind is the body, and the subtle part of the body is the mind, like the yin-yang symbol. This perspective makes it easier to unravel the intricate body-mind connection. We are familiar with psychosomatic illness, where beliefs, habits, attitudes, and emotions manifest physically. But have you ever thought about the reverse? Disturbances in the body—especially those related to the gut, inflammation, nutritional deficiencies, or hormonal imbalances—create havoc far more dangerous than the psychosomatic connection.

Consider the gut-brain axis. The gut, often called the "second brain," houses a vast network of neurons and produces neurotransmitters, just like the brain. When the gut is disturbed—whether through inflammation, infection, or poor diet—it sends distress signals to the brain, leading to changes in mood, cognition, and behavior. Conditions like Irritable Bowel Syndrome (IBS) and Small Intestinal Bacterial Overgrowth (SIBO) are linked to anxiety and depression, illustrating this powerful connection.

But it's not all about the bad bacteria. Our gut is home to trillions of good bacteria, collectively known as the microbiome. These beneficial microbes play a crucial role in maintaining our health. They aid digestion, produce essential vitamins, and protect against harmful pathogens. More importantly, they help regulate our immune system and influence our mental health. A healthy microbiome produces neurotransmitters like serotonin, often dubbed the "feel-good" hormone, which significantly affects our mood and overall mental well-being. Disruptions in the microbiome balance, known as dysbiosis, can lead to inflammation and increased intestinal permeability, often referred to as "leaky gut." This condition allows toxins and bacteria to enter the bloodstream, potentially affecting the brain and contributing to a fractured mind.

"Have you ever stopped to wonder how deeply connected your body and mind truly are? Imagine a small fire smoldering quietly within—a fire meant to warm and sustain life. But what happens when that fire grows unchecked, fueled by unhealthy habits, stress, or poor nourishment? This is chronic inflammation: a silent blaze that begins in the body but soon sends its smoke signals to the brain.

The body's immune system, meant to protect, ends up overreacting, releasing inflammatory cytokines—tiny messengers of distress. These messengers do not respect boundaries; they cross the blood-brain barrier and disrupt the intricate symphony of the mind. Neurotransmitters, the brain's instruments of mood and cognition, falter. The result? A mind weighed down by depression, anxiety, or a fog that clouds every thought.

And then there's the quiet hunger beneath it all—nutritional deficiencies that sap vitality from within. Vitamins like B12 and D, and minerals such as magnesium and zinc, are not just nutrients; they are lifelines for the brain. Without them, the mind struggles, like a plant deprived of sunlight, wilting into depression or cognitive decline.

But it is not just about the food we eat or the nutrients we lack. It is about balance, harmony—within the body's own orchestra of hormones. The endocrine system, with its delicate threads of connection, regulates not just your physical state but your emotional landscape as well. When this balance tips the mind feels the ripple effects: anxiety, depression, even the erosion of memory and focus.

The liver, a silent sentinel of the body, works tirelessly to cleanse and purify. It filters out harmful substances, ensuring the blood that courses through us remains life-giving. But what happens when the liver, overburdened or sluggish, falters in its task? Toxins accumulate—heavy metals, metabolic byproducts, even neurotoxins like ammonia—escaping the liver's grasp and traveling to the brain. Their presence disrupts neurotransmitters, muddles thought processes, and clouds emotional clarity, creating an inner storm.

This toxic build-up manifests in the body as sleeplessness, which is often the first crack in the system. Sleeplessness invites a torrent of unstoppable thoughts, stiffened nerves, and a body trapped in survival mode. The sympathetic nervous system kicks in, gearing us for fight-or-flight, a mechanism designed for brief danger. But when prolonged, this state becomes an internal siege—heart racing, mind alert but not clear, body hyperaroused yet exhausted.

Sleep, our natural reset, becomes elusive. The lack of it further blurs cognitive clarity, disrupts mood regulation, and deepens emotional instability. As sleeplessness festers, anger brews, erupting as harsh words or impulsive actions. Relationships strain, thoughts fragment, and the mind feels caught in a tug-of-war between the body's distress and the brain's search for equilibrium.

I call this state the fractured mind. Fractured because it is torn—pulled apart by physical imbalance and mental chaos. But fractures, as nature shows us, are not irreparable. Just as a broken bone mends with care, so too can the fractured mind heal.

Healing begins by addressing the body, the mind's foundation. Proper nutrition—whole foods, fresh fruits, and nutrient-rich vegetables—supports the liver and brain alike. Sunshine, often overlooked, is a free healer; 15 minutes in natural light recharges the mind and strengthens the body. Barefoot walks on the earth ground us, reconnecting the fragmented parts of our being.

Movement, particularly stretches and rhythmic activities like yoga, dance, or mindful walking, holds profound healing power. These practices stimulate the lymphatic system, our body's waste disposal network. Unlike the circulatory system, which has the heart's rhythmic pulse, the lymphatic system relies on muscle movement and deep breathing. Each stretch and inhale become an act of cleansing, a step toward restoring the body's natural balance.

And balance is everything. When the body finds balance, the mind follows. Breathing deeply floods the brain with oxygen, restoring severed neural connections and quieting the chaos. Stretching expands not just the muscles but also the mind, allowing it to move beyond the confines of distress. Slowly, the fractured mind begins to piece itself together.

In this healing process, the connection between body and mind reveals itself as a delicate dance—bidirectional and profound. When one falters, the other wavers. When one heals, the other follows. Understanding this interplay and caring for both is the path to not just survival but true vitality. The fractured mind, though broken, holds within it the blueprint for healing.

Understanding the interconnectedness of the body and mind opens the door to examining broader influences on our mental well-being. While physiological and lifestyle factors play a crucial role, social and environmental elements are equally significant in shaping mental health. This brings us to Johann Hari's illuminating perspectives on the hidden costs of medication.

The Hidden Costs of Medication: Insights from Johann Hari

In *Lost Connections,* Johann Hari explores the idea that rising rates of depression and anxiety are not merely the result of chemical imbalances in the brain but are deeply rooted in a range of social and environmental factors. He argues that while antidepressant medications can provide temporary relief for some, they often fail to address the root causes of mental health issues and come with significant side effects.

Hari's main critique of antidepressant medications is that they often lead to dependency and can have diminishing returns over time. He highlights studies showing that, although these medications can be effective for some individuals, they frequently fail to outperform placebos in many cases. Furthermore, he points out that such medications can cause side effects like weight gain, sexual dysfunction, and emotional numbness, all of which can further erode a person's quality of life.

As a solution, Hari advocates for a more holistic approach to mental health, emphasizing the need to address the underlying causes of depression and anxiety. He identifies nine key factors contributing to mental distress:

1. Disconnection from Meaningful Work: Engaging in fulfilling work can significantly improve mental health.

2. Disconnection from Other People: Building strong, supportive relationships is crucial for emotional well-being.

3. Disconnection from Meaningful Values: Living in alignment with personal values and beliefs can provide a sense of purpose and direction.

4. Disconnection from Childhood Trauma: Addressing and healing past traumas is vital for overcoming long-term emotional pain.

5. Disconnection from Status and Respect: Feeling valued and respected within a community or social structure is important for self-esteem.

6. Disconnection from the Natural World: Spending time in nature has been shown to reduce stress and improve mood.

7. Disconnection from a Secure Future: Economic and social stability are essential for reducing anxiety and fostering a sense of security.

8. Role of Genes and Brain Changes: While acknowledging biology's role, Hari argues that it is often overemphasized at the expense of addressing social factors.

9. Disconnection from a Hopeful or Secure Future: Addressing societal and economic factors that contribute to a sense of hopelessness is key.

As we consider Hari's holistic approach to mental health, we see that he not only advocates for individual healing practices but also for societal changes. These include policies that promote economic security, social justice, and community building. On an individual level, he encourages people to engage in activities that foster connection, purpose, and emotional healing. This includes therapy, community involvement, meaningful work, and lifestyle changes that promote both physical and mental well-being.

Reflecting on the journey of the twin sisters who overcame their own mental health challenges, the lesson is clear: Respond, do not react.

CHAPTER 8

THE SOIL AND THE WEEDS: A LESSON IN TRUE HEALING

As the sun began its descent, the garden seemed to hold its breath, enveloped in a serene stillness. The gentle rustling of leaves and the soft chirping of birds created a melody that blended seamlessly with the setting. It was a stark contrast to the hurried pace of life beyond these walls, a sanctuary where thoughts could finally settle. Recollections of our previous thoughts on balance felt natural here, as though the garden itself whispered the wisdom of slowing down and listening deeply.

I found myself pacing along the stone pathway, my thoughts heavier than the calm around me. The Wise Healer sat cross-legged on a weathered bench, his eyes calm yet observant, following my restless steps. Finally, I paused mid-step, looking around and taking in the tranquility. "It's so peaceful here, Master," I remarked, lowering myself to sit on the grass. A sigh escaped me as I added, "The world outside feels so chaotic in comparison."

The Healer's faint smile carried the weight of understanding. "Peace is not about the absence of chaos," he said, his voice steady, "but the ability to remain still amidst it. What troubles your mind today?"

"It's health," I admitted. "I have been thinking about what it truly means. Modern medicine boasts about cures, yet people are still sick. Diabetes, heart disease, even simple eyesight problems—they call it 'management,' not 'cure.' Isn't health supposed to mean freedom from all of it?"

The Healer's expression softened, his tone calm but firm. "Take a deep breath. Your mind is like the wind—always moving, never still. No truth is clear when the wind stirs the water."

I frowned slightly but complied, the breath steadying me. "Fine. But I need clarity, not riddles. Why do we call something a 'cure' or 'treatment' when the disease returns? Is modern medicine lying to us?"

He chuckled, a gentle sound that did not dismiss the question but eased its weight. "No, they are not lying," he said. "But they are limited by their way of seeing. Treatment is just addressing the symptoms to relieve pain. The root cause is not addressed. Imagine a man with weeds in his garden. Modern medicine pulls out the weeds, even sprays them with chemicals. For a time, the garden appears clean. Pulling out the weeds is the cure, while spraying is the treatment."

I nodded in understanding, but a troubling thought lingered: "But the roots remain. The weeds grow back." The Healer responded, "Exactly. The cure and treatment are surface level. They address the visible, the measurable, the tangible. But healing... healing is different." Intrigued, I leaned forward, "How so?" The Healer explained, "Healing is about transforming the soil. It asks, 'Why did the weeds grow in the first place?' Was the soil poor? Too much water? Too much sun? Healing is not about fighting the weeds but restoring balance so that weeds no longer have a reason to grow." This made me think, so if I understand correctly, a 'cure' is when you remove the problem. But 'healing' is about changing the environment, so the problem doesn't come back." The Healer nodded, "Yes, but go deeper. Cure is an act; it is done to the body. Healing is a process; it happens within the person. A cure focuses on the disease. Healing focuses on the person. Do you see the difference?"

Thinking aloud, I responded, "So when a doctor gives me antibiotics to kill bacteria, that's a cure. But if I keep eating poorly and weakening my immune system, I will get sick again. No healing has taken place." The Healer affirmed, "Yes. You have learned well. This is why people can be 'cured' of cancer but remain in fear of its return. Their bodies are fixed, but their minds are still broken. Healing, true healing reaches beyond the physical. It touches the emotional, mental, and spiritual dimensions of a person." Hesitantly, I asked, "What about chronic conditions like diabetes or vision problems? People do not actually get completely cured from those, do they?"

The Healer's eyes narrowed, his voice firm, "Yes. Diseases like cancer, diabetes, and heart disease cannot be cured completely; they can only be managed according to modern health care. All these diseases are like dormant volcanoes. They erupt when there is a lapse on the part of the beholder when there is no transformation from within. On the other hand, healing is all about holistic well-being." I was confused but curious, "But how can one bring about this transformation and what is this holistic well-being?" The Healer explained, "Transformation begins with a yearning to know yourself completely in and out. Trusting your body that it can heal itself when given the right internal environment the way soil replenishes its nutrients with the right water, air, and sunshine." I leaned forward, straightening my posture, intrigued, "This is interesting… please continue."

The Healer continued, "And your next question was about holistic healing. Holistic means becoming whole as opposed to being fragmented. It is the restoration of harmony and balance. If you learn to live in balance with your body's needs—in food, rest, thought, and spirit; live according to the Circadian rhythms, aligned with Nature, then you are on your way to holistic healing." I leaned back, my eyes widening in realization, "So even if I'm not 'cured' of something, I can still be healed." The Healer nodded slowly, "Yes. And you must see that the world's obsession with 'cures' is why so many are still unhealed. They chase pills, surgeries, and quick fixes. They uproot weeds but never tend to the soil. Their bodies are patched up, but their hearts remain restless, their minds full of doubt." Thoughtful,

I reflected, "So… cure is like maintenance. Fix it when it breaks. But healing is like preventive care—tend to the soil before the weeds even grow."

The Healer smiled deeply, "Ah, you have seen it. In the Quran, this is called taqwa—awareness, caution, foresight. You do not wait for the storm to come before you shelter your house. You strengthen it before the winds arrive. Healing is foresight, not reaction." My voice filled with realization, "This is why you say healing is across four dimensions. Physical is just one part. If I only 'cure' my body but leave my mind full of thoughts, my emotions full of fear and anger, and my spirit disconnected, unsatisfied without peace, I'm still broken." The Healer responded, "Yes, child. True healing happens when you recognize that you are not just a body with parts to be fixed. You are a whole being. Your thoughts affect your heart, your heart affects your organs, and your organs affect your mind. You are not separate pieces. You are one." I smiled faintly, "I see now. Cure is for the body—incomplete, but healing is for the self—holistic." The Healer's eyes softened, "Yes. And when you understand that you will no longer fear disease. You will see it as a message, a teacher, a guide. You would have moved from disease to Ease." I looked at the horizon, "This changes everything, Master. The world says, 'Remove the problem,' but you say, 'Restore the balance.'"

The Healer, gazing at the sunset, affirmed, "Yes, child. Disease is not your enemy. It is the body's voice calling you back to balance. Do not silence it with quick fixes. Listen. Learn. Heal." That was enlightening. His every step hummed with intention—not the careful tread of the old, but the quiet certainty of roots pressing deeper into the earth. The sun caught the silver in his hair, but his face bore only whispers of time, not its heavy grip. His eyes, though, told another story—depths where decades had pooled, like rainwater gathered in a stone basin.

I had placed him in his 60s, may be 65 if I was being unkind. But as he reached for a sprig of herbs from the garden, he glanced at me, his smile slow but sharp. "When you've seen ninety-three seasons," he said, his eyes glinting like the edge of a blade, "you learn not to rush."

"What?" I stammered, the weight of that number filling the air around us, thicker than mist after rain. Ninety-three? My mind struggled to reconcile the number with the man before me—his movements fluid, his gaze alive with clarity, his energy unyielding. "How?" I blurted out, the question slipping from my lips before I could catch it. "How do you... stay like this?"

Crushing the herb leaves between his fingers, releasing their fragrance into the air, he spoke steadily, "Healing is not about fighting time, but aligning with it. The body, the mind, the spirit—they are not meant to rush ahead or linger behind. They're meant to move in harmony, like the seasons." Turning to me and holding up the crushed leaves, he continued, "Do you see these herbs? They grow not by force, but by rhythm—by trusting the cycles of the sun, the rain, the soil. We are no different. When you align with the rhythms of your body, your emotions, your thoughts, and the world around you, you stop aging in the way people think of it. You don't freeze time, but you live in its flow, unburdened by its weight."

I nodded slowly, still processing his words. "So healing is... balance?"

"Balance, yes," he said, his gaze steady, "and respect. Respect for the seasons of life, for the signals your body sends, for the connections that sustain you. When you fight against time or nature, you age faster. But when you align with them, you grow—stronger, deeper, like roots pressing into the earth. That is how you truly heal."

His words hung in the air, settling into me like seeds ready to take root. I watched as he walked away, his steps steady as the ticking of a clock—not one that chased hours, but one that marked the rhythm of a life fully aligned. Silence fell as the sun dipped below the horizon, casting a golden glow over the garden. My mind was still, but no longer restless. The water of the mind had stilled.

KNOW THYSELF

From the profound stillness of the garden where insights into healing were shared, the journey of understanding deepens. The words "Know Thyself" are etched on the walls of the Academy founded by the great philosopher Plato, a student of Socrates, and I was so awed by these words which at first did not make any sense. "Mr. Parvez, through his enlightening books, introduced me to these Greek philosophers. Their wisdom, now part of our intellectual heritage, sparked a lifelong passion for philosophy in me."

As I reflected on the concept of 'Know Thyself,' I realized that it was not just a philosophical mantra, but a guiding principle to my work as a healer. Moreover, I saw how this idea echoed in the Quran verse, 'they also are at peace with what was revealed before you.' This connection led me to understand that true healing requires a holistic approach, one that acknowledges the interconnectedness of body, mind, emotions, and spirit. Furthermore, I began to see how this understanding could transform my relationships with patients, moving beyond just treating symptoms to addressing the whole person.

So, following in the footsteps of these philosophers, the first question they asked and sought to answer was "Who am I?" As a healer, I ask the same questions to those who come to me with their ailments because knowing oneself not only empowers individuals to heal but also transforms their lives. Their answers: I am my body, I am my mind, I am my emotions, some tend to go deep and say I am the life force, meaning the vital spirit that shuts off at death.

I often tell my patients, "You are partly right but also missing the larger truth. You are not merely your body, mind, emotions, or spirit; you are an integrated whole—these elements do not exist separately but interdependently. Therefore, to heal, you must first journey inward and know yourself."

One thing is common among most people: they dwell only on those things that demand immediate attention. In other words, they believe in breakdown maintenance. Perennial wisdom in the Quran, on the other hand, stresses being cautious, i.e., preventive maintenance. This concept assumes that you have prior knowledge of the transaction you are about to undertake, including the possibilities of what may go wrong, or the dangers involved in the pathway.

So, the first step toward healing is to know your body—its anatomy, the dashboard, the physical dimension; your mind—its thoughts, aptitudes, attitudes, beliefs, habits, desires, and memories—the mental dimension; your feelings—ranging from happiness to pride, irritation to anger, envy to jealousy, and the ability to manage and resolve them—the emotional dimension; and the ability to understand your connection with creation and the vital force that runs through this universe, surrendering yourself to something larger than you, whether God, nature, or society—the spiritual dimension.

A cell is the fundamental unit of the human body, just as a brick is the fundamental unit of a building. A group of cells forms a tissue. A group of tissues forms an organ. A group of organs forms a system, and the entire system becomes the human organism. In other words, approximately 100 trillion cells work together in synchrony and unison as one single human organism—that is you. To understand the nature of the human body, it is enough to understand the workings of a single cell. The microcosm is the macrocosm, and creation mimics the universe in miniature. Have you not witnessed how billions of years of evolutionary drama are frozen and shrunk in the womb, unfolding from a single-cell zygote to a fully grown human baby?

The basic function of any cell, tissue, organ, or the body is digestion. Assimilation and elimination are the two functions of digestion. Though they appear as two functions, they are the same, fused together like the Yin and Yang symbol. The end part of assimilation is elimination; the starting point of elimination is assimilation.

Similarly, respiration involves inhaling and exhaling, blinking is the closing and opening of eyes, and a heartbeat is contraction and expansion. All these are two characteristics of one function, like day and night, cold and hot, rising and falling, male and female. Each one complements the other and is incomplete without the other.

Why do the cells perform this function? To live! This answers the toughest philosophical question simply. Truth is always simple, but humans complicate it. Energy—the life force—is necessary to sustain life. We need air, water, and food to produce this energy. Assimilation involves absorbing the nutrients contained in air, water, and food. The process that extracts the energy generates morbid matter or waste, meaning the process to get energy has waste generation built into it.

The energy thus obtained is utilized as:

1. Digestive energy

2. Functional energy

3. Maintenance energy

Functional energy is needed for involuntary functions of all internal organs and voluntary functions such as the movement of limbs, seeing, hearing, talking, and smelling.

Eat when Hungry;
Drink when Thirsty;
Rest when Sleepy.

"When you over-do under-do or
do not do timely Disease sets in"

Digestive energy is especially important in the sense that it not only consumes the energy needed to digest the food but is also responsible for replenishing the same energy. If digestion is improper, the energy required by the entire body suffers. Both functional and maintenance energy rely on this digestive energy.

Maintenance energy, also known as immune or restorative energy, ensures that both functional and digestive energies produce waste in the body. Immune energy safely removes these wastes without disturbing the normal functioning of the body.

In the normal functioning of the body, energy is equally distributed among the three functions at approximately 33% each. The body is said to be in harmony with natural laws—eating when hungry, drinking when thirsty, and sleeping or resting at proper times, as demanded by the body.

When a deer grazes and suddenly senses danger from a predator, its sympathetic nervous system springs into action, triggering a host of chemical reactions within its body, and the deer runs for its life. Once the deer is far from danger, its body relaxes and returns to its original, normal state.

Humans, however, often remain in a perpetual fight-or-flight mode even after the danger has passed, primarily due to constant dwelling on thoughts. Imagine our energy being continuously consumed by dwelling on incidents from the past or imaginary anxieties about the future. The mind cannot differentiate between the actual and the imaginary—both play out in the same manner on the screen of our consciousness.

When the body is perpetually in an emergency mode, energy is not available for the immune system, which is essential to fight diseases ranging from the common cold to cancer. Our body is designed to tackle such challenges, provided the required energy is available. This is why, when we are sick, we often don't feel like eating or moving much—the immune system takes over, redirecting digestive and functional energy to where it's needed most.

This remarkable ability to prioritize and heal itself is a testament to the profound intelligence within our bodies—a tireless wisdom that operates beyond our conscious awareness and deserves our trust in its rightful place.

Trust Your Body

Body heals itself but in its time. Therefore wait patiently. When you speed up with medicines & surgery you are interfering with its inherent healing properties and biological rhythm. Now the body has to deal with intervention and set right its house simultaneously. Most of the time our body endures but with repeated assaults it gives up.

As we reflect on the body's remarkable ability to prioritize and heal itself, it becomes clear that this wisdom extends far beyond our conscious control. You didn't teach your body to breathe, to start your heartbeat, or to digest food—it all happens naturally, without effort. Yet, when it comes to healing, many of us race from one remedy to the next, believing that a cure requires constant action or external treatment. This mindset reflects two different perspectives: one that stays open to new ideas and exploration, and another that clings to existing beliefs, leaving no room for growth.

To those who are closed-minded, I often say: "Experience is the ultimate teacher, but wisdom lies in learning from others' experiences." Wise individuals do not always need to endure the pain of trial and error to discover the truth—they observe, listen, and take note of the outcome others have had. It is vital to question everything, even the most sacred ideas, and to remain discerning. Do not be too quick to accept things as they are—there is always more to learn and understand.

The body itself offers countless examples of self-healing, proving that many processes are already built into us, requiring nothing more than trust and balance. Consider how, when you cut your finger or fall and hurt yourself, the body at once clots the blood, forming a protective mesh around the wound to prevent further blood loss. Even before you can apply an ointment, the wound begins to heal, covered by a new layer of skin. The initial loss of blood serves another purpose—it prevents foreign particles from entering the body, reducing contamination to a minimum. This lays down the golden rule: the body does not allow anything beneficial to escape nor anything harmful to enter.

This is the inherent intelligence of the body, a timeless wisdom that silently safeguards our well-being.

When an expectant mother completes her nine months, pain automatically develops and starts pushing the baby. Even with an abortion for some reason, if the fetus inside stops developing, the body pushes out the undeveloped fetus. Who performs this act? The body's primal need is its own survival.

Children, when they bang themselves against a wall or fall, develop swelling around the area of impact, accompanied by pain. This swelling results from the increased movement of fluid and white blood cells to the injured area. The release of chemicals and the compression of nerves in injury cause pain. Pain and swelling are inherent mechanisms that keep the body from using the injured part, protecting it from further injury.

When a bone fractures, the fracture is naturally filled by a process called calcification, a natural healing process initiated by the body.

Once the mother delivers the baby, the breast is ready with milk for the newborn. This arrangement is natural and to date, there has not been a more nutritious and healthy drink that not only nourishes but also strengthens the immune system of the newborn. The body is self-sufficient.

Labour pain brings out a Baby;
Stomach pain eliminates faeces;

"Pain anywhere signifies
Movement & Removal of Toxins – A
Harbinger of Ease."

Certain actions of the body are so obvious and taken for granted that we often do not stop to consider how the body carries out this. Sleep is the best healing mechanism. Detoxification only occurs during sleep, as it has its own mechanism for overhauling and detoxing.

If there is food poisoning or indigestion, the body expels the food, preventing further damage to the entire system either through vomit or dysentery. With minimal energy spent, the body provides maximum comfort without disturbing the vital functions of breathing, blood circulation, and excretion.

These examples illustrate the remarkable ability of the body to self-regulate and heal, underscoring the wisdom of trusting in its innate mechanisms to maintain health and restore balance.

CHAPTER 10

HEALING ACROSS FOUR DIMENSIONS

The wisdom of the body to self-regulate and heal, as explored in the previous chapter, lays the foundation for understanding the deeper layers of human well-being. Beyond the physical processes of repair and renewal, healing encompasses a profound interplay of the body, mind, emotions, and spirit. This seamless integration is not just about addressing symptoms but about achieving harmony across all aspects of our being.

I prefer the word heal over cure because it conveys a sense of wholeness—a state where the entire organism actively participates in maintaining balance, well-being, and ease. Healing is not a linear process confined to one part of the body or mind; it is a symphony of interactions within us. To help explain this concept more clearly, I have identified four dimensions of healing: Physical, Emotional, Mental, and Spiritual. The way you act, think, and feel reveals the interplay of these dimensions.

Actions are tied to the Physical Dimension, thoughts to the Mental Dimension, but feelings?

Feelings straddle two realms, requiring discernment. When feelings are wholesome—rooted in contentment, gratitude, compassion, and empathy—they belong to the Spiritual Dimension. These are feelings that uplift, expand, and connect you to the essence of life itself. But when feelings waver—rising and falling like turbulent waves, leaving you drained and weary— they align with the Emotional Dimension. These feelings, though vital, are more transient and reactive, reflecting the ebb and flow of human experience. The Spiritual Dimension serves as the core, the vital life force interwoven with every cell of the body, subtler than the mind yet profoundly powerful. It doesn't stand apart from the other dimensions but permeates them all, like water saturating the fibers of a sponge. Recognizing which dimension you are operating from requires awareness—a conscious tuning into the nuances of your inner world.

Similarly, there is a distinction between inspiration and thoughts, though both arise on the conscious plane. How can you differentiate them? The nature of their content holds the answer. Thoughts are often selfish, seeking instant gratification or immediate resolution. They are tied to personal desires and fleeting concerns. Inspirations, however, come from a higher plane. They are selfless, offering solutions not just for the individual but for the greater good. Inspirations spark ideas for invention, revelations that transform lives, and discoveries that serve humanity.

"Do a minor correction in the Spiritual Dimension before it manifests as a lifestyle disease in the Physical Dimension"

Understanding this subtle difference can guide you to align your actions, thoughts, and feelings with the higher dimensions, allowing you to experience life as a harmonious whole rather than a fragmented struggle. The Physical dimension serves us like the dashboard of our car that shows speed, fuel, temperature, and oil. Symptoms of discomfort, weakness, pain, and nausea are the markers of this dimension. It is only through this dimension that we take corrective action by changing the way we breathe, eat food, drink water, and sleep at appropriate times. Twenty-five percent of the problem is solved.

To explore the practical application of these dimensions further, I turned to Shams, a holistic teacher whose insights bridge ancient wisdom with modern science. During my interview with Shams, I shared my personal health experiences, from childhood to my school days. Like any other child, I encountered the usual colds, flu, coughs, and fevers. I vividly remember suffering from typhoid and malaria attacks that lasted 1-2 weeks. Back then, the general advice from elders was, "A controlled diet speeds up recovery." At the time, I did not pay much attention, but now, at 58, I view their advice as wisdom, patiently waiting for years for someone to truly apply and benefit from it. Indeed, with my own body as both the subject and the object of this experiment—proving that our bodies can heal themselves—I confidently affirm that "Food Should Be Our Medicine."

He said, "I am glad that you are living the knowledge you have gathered across your journey of life aligned with nature. The aphorism 'Food is medicine' is from one of our ancient Siddha sages of Tamil Nadu. They have spent their lives observing nature and humans. It is not as simple as it sounds. It's an ocean in a drop. It has various aspects to it: what to eat, what not to eat, how much to eat, when to eat, whether to eat fresh or cooked, and the quantity one should eat. It's more than eating etiquette."

The best food is what nature provides us in the form of fruits, vegetables, nuts, whole grains, and millets. Uncooked and unprocessed, most of them are alkaline. They create an environment of regeneration and reduce oxidative stress. In an acidic state, there is fatigue, inflammation, bone demineralization, and a weak immune system. Not that an acidic state is unwanted—the stomach requires an acidic state for digestion—but the body maintains the pH balance and requires a slightly alkaline state to function efficiently. This, in simple terms, means cells become healthier and rust-free. Semi-cooked food, i.e., boiled and baked, has a lower nutritional value because cooking blurs the data stored in the food. Our body's enzymes are not able to read the information contained in the food we eat when it is cooked for too long.[1]

---

1   *   pH is a scale that measures how acidic or alkaline something is, from 0 to 14.
- 0–6 is acidic (like lemon juice or vinegar).
- 7 is neutral (like pure water).
- 8–14 is alkaline (like baking soda or seawater).

In the body, we aim for a slightly alkaline balance to stay healthy, with blood pH around 7.4. Too much acidity or alkalinity can cause health problems, so the body works hard to keep it just right.

This balance is not limited to just physical processes but extends to how we nourish our entire being. Shams observed, "The aphorism isn't limited to just physical food; it speaks to all that we take in through our senses. What we see, hear, touch, taste, and even think becomes a form of nourishment for the body, mind, and spirit. Everything we experience feeds us, shaping our energy and influencing our inner state. Just as the food we consume affects our health, the images we witness, the sounds we listen to, and the thoughts we entertain shape our well-being."

"For every input, there is an output," Shams continued. "The output of the food we consume is energy and residue—the way ash is produced after burning wood. This energy, what we call functional energy, is expressed in the form of movement, thoughts, and emotions. Talking about emotions, feelings serve as the stamp of awareness, marking how you experience life. Just as the tongue discerns the taste and texture of food, feelings reveal the texture and tone of an experience, offering insight into its meaning and outcomes."

"Remember, what we consume through senses is food, and what consumes us are emotions. And do not forget, emotion is energy in motion. I will end this day with food for thought. Mull over. Tomorrow we will discuss this idea."

These words forged a deep connection between the tangible and the intangible, emphasizing that everything we take in—be it food, sights, or thoughts—shapes both our inner balance and outer well-being.

Here is a glimpse of what unfolded the next day.

"Yesterday, you said what we consume through the senses is food, and what consumes us are our emotions," I began, still puzzled but sensing a deeper meaning. "At first, I didn't understand, but now I think there's something more. Can you explain?" Shams nodded, explaining, "That statement introduces the Emotional Dimension. Emotions are energy in motion, carrying messages about your boundaries, values, and needs. When you breathe deeply and consciously, you allow this energy to flow and transform. However, shallow, unmindful breathing traps emotions, creating stagnation and dis-ease." I pondered his words, then asked, "And when you said emotions consume us, what does that mean?" Shams replied, "Emotions give expression to energy. Like food, they too need a small amount of energy to metabolize. But when emotions are not examined for their genuineness or usefulness, they can overwhelm you—like an unchecked fire. They consume us."

Intrigued, I reflected, "So emotions are like fire—capable of warming or destroying, depending on how

Be Conscious of:

What you Eat,
What you Feel,
What you Think,
What you Believe,

Your Physical, Emotional, Mental &
Spiritual Health is Taken Care of.

we manage them?" "Exactly," Shams affirmed. "Fire can light the way or destroy everything. Similarly, emotions must be channeled wisely. If anger, fear, or sadness takes over, it consumes you. But when understood, emotions become a source of strength and creativity." "How can we channel emotions instead of letting them consume us?" I asked, eager to learn more.

"Through awareness," Shams advised. "When an emotion arises, don't suppress or run from it—both reactions only add to its weight. Instead, pause and acknowledge it for what it is: energy in motion, a messenger carrying valuable information. Ask yourself: What is this emotion telling me? What boundary, need, or value does it reflect? Then, consciously choose how to direct its energy constructively." He continued, "For instance, imagine you're feeling anger. Instead of snapping at someone or bottling it up, take a moment to breathe and reflect. Anger often points to a perceived injustice or a boundary that has been crossed. Ask: What triggered this anger? Is it something within my control? If the anger stems from being overburdened at work, perhaps it's telling you to set clearer boundaries or voice your needs.

Instead of lashing out, channel that energy into a calm but firm conversation with your manager or a colleague: "I have noticed my workload has increased significantly. Can we discuss a way to manage this better?" By acknowledging and redirecting the energy of anger, you not only address the issue at its root but also prevent it from festering or escalating into resentment or burnout. Similarly, sadness may appear as a sign of unacknowledged loss or a longing for connection. Instead of pushing it aside, lean into the emotion. Reflect: What am I grieving? What do I need to feel whole again? This could lead you to reach out to a loved one for support or take time to honor what you have lost through journaling or a personal ritual. When emotions are met with awareness, they become guides rather than obstacles. They point the way toward healing, growth, and greater alignment with your true self.

"So, emotions aren't the problem—it's how we relate to them?" I asked.

"Precisely," Shams replied. "Emotions are messengers. Fear warns of danger, joy signals alignment, anger calls for justice, and sadness invites release. When you understand them, they enrich your life force. When ignored, they create chaos."

"It's like choosing the right food—both nourish us when managed wisely," I added.

"Yes," Shams said, nodding. "Both food and emotions shape your energy. When you master what you consume and how you process it, you align with life's rhythm. No longer consumed by chaos, you flow like a river, bringing nourishment to yourself and others."

I reflected for a moment before continuing, "I've worked through the physical and emotional dimensions, but now it's time to tackle the mental dimension. What does healing here involve?"

"The mental dimension is like the control tower of your life," Shams explained. "It governs your beliefs, attitudes, habits, memories, and thoughts. These are the filters through which you perceive the world and the patterns that guide your choices."

"Beliefs… That is a big one," I said thoughtfully. "How do they fit into healing?"

"Your beliefs are the foundation of your mental world," Shams began. "They shape what you see as possible and impossible. Healing here means uncovering the beliefs that limit you and replacing them with those that empower you. Ask yourself: Does this belief support the life I want to live? If not, it's time to let it go."

"But why are we so attached to our beliefs?" I asked.

"It's because they are like our possessions—material possessions that can make us feel good and secure," Shams explained. "Even the way we talk about beliefs is similar to how we talk about things we own. We 'hold,' 'acquire,' 'inherit,' and 'give up' beliefs. But our beliefs are more than possessions—they are part of our very identity. Criticism of our beliefs can feel like a criticism of ourselves."

"To stretch out your Mind so that it loosens
the grip of its beliefs that are latched onto it,
stretch your body with focus on your breath;
The beliefs would drop like smithereens"

"Ah, how true!" I exclaimed. "I now recall two pivotal moments in my life that elevated me to a higher pedestal. One was about my belief in God, and the other about health. I had a very narrow view of the Creator—somewhere up in the sky, single, powerful—but after reading the Quran, my perspective shifted profoundly. It revealed a dynamic Creator, deeply infused, and involved with creation, operating through unchanging laws. I began to see manifestations of beauty, balance, harmony, and peace throughout nature, continuously evolving. This understanding moved me away from anthropomorphic inclinations toward a more expansive, interconnected, all-inclusive view of the Divine—an energy whose qualities we are meant to embody and replicate at every possible human level."

Realizing the freedom and expansiveness I gained from questioning my belief about how I perceived God, I continued, "I began to question everything I had taken for granted. This led to another shift in my perspective on health—I came to trust the body's innate ability to heal itself, recognizing that any interference not aligned with natural laws is a form of blasphemy."

"Thank you for your patience… About attitudes? How are they different from beliefs?" I asked.

Shams replied, "If beliefs are the foundation, attitudes are the lens. They color your view of life—positive or negative, open, or closed. A healing attitude is one of curiosity and gratitude, especially in the face of challenges. It's about seeing obstacles not as barriers, but as steppingstones."

"That sounds easier said than done," I admitted. "How do I change a deeply ingrained attitude?"

"Start small," Shams advised. "Each day, look for one thing to appreciate, even in difficulty. Over time, gratitude rewires the mind. Healing doesn't demand giant leaps—it thrives in consistent, gentle shifts."

"What about habits?" I asked. "They seem more about actions than the mind."

Shams nodded. "Mental habits are the routines of thought that run on autopilot—like overthinking, procrastination, or self-criticism. Healing means recognizing these patterns and replacing them with healthier ones. Think of it like tending a garden. Weed out what doesn't serve you and nurture what does."

"That makes sense," I said. "And memories? They feel so deeply rooted—how can they be healed?"

"Memories are the stories you carry, but they don't have to define you," Shams explained. "Painful memories, if left unhealed, can trap you in the past. But when you reframe them—as lessons rather than wounds—they transform into guides. Healing begins when you stop resisting the past and start learning from it."

"Thoughts must be the most constant part of this dimension," I mused. "How do they fit into the healing process?"

"Thoughts are the seeds of your reality," Shams said. "They can create clarity or chaos. Healing the mind means cultivating awareness of your thoughts—choosing which to nourish and which to release. Silence and stillness, through practices like meditation or journaling, are your greatest allies."

"So healing the mental dimension is really about gaining mastery over these ingredients?" I asked, beginning to piece it all together.

"Exactly," Shams affirmed. "Mastery—not control. When you understand the role of attitudes, habits, memories, and thoughts, and align them with your deeper self, you gain the clarity to navigate life's complexities with ease and purpose."

"Yes, mastery—not control. When you stop being ruled by your beliefs, attitudes, habits, memories, and thoughts, you become the architect of your inner world. This alignment is the bridge from mental chaos to mental clarity, from dis-ease to ease," explained Shams.

"And when the mind aligns, do the other dimensions follow?" I inquired.

"The mind is the thread that connects the physical, emotional, and spiritual dimensions. Heal the mental, and the rest will harmonize. Let your thoughts guide you, not bind you," Shams responded.

"Thank you. I will start tending this garden, one belief, one attitude, and one thought at a time," I affirmed.

"And as you do, remember—what you plant in the mind blooms in your life. Choose wisely, and let it grow with purpose and peace. Beware! Every thought ends in a biological fact," Shams cautioned.

"Wow! This is too deep," I exclaimed.

"Yes, and that's why thoughts are so powerful. But let me ask you this: where do these thoughts originate?" Shams posed the question.

"From the mind, of course," I replied.

"True, but the mind doesn't act in isolation. Its thoughts are shaped by something deeper—an underlying force that guides, nourishes, and sustains it," Shams elucidated.

"You're talking about the core or vital spirit you keep mentioning, aren't you?" I asked.

"The core is the unseen essence of who you are. While the mind translates its messages into thoughts, habits, and beliefs, the core is the source—the pure, unchanging center that holds the blueprint for your well-being and growth," Shams elaborated.

"So, the core is where it all begins?" I sought confirmation.

*"Beware A Thought Ends
in a Biological Fact."*

"Yes. It's the source of inspiration, intuition, and alignment. And just as every thought becomes a biological fact, the messages from the core shape your entire being—if you're open to receiving them," Shams concluded, introducing the Spiritual Dimension.

"You often speak of the core as if it holds all the answers. What exactly is the core?" I pondered.

"The core, or what some might call the vital spirit, is the very essence of Nature within us. It's not just a part of you—it's a representative of the entirety of Nature, holding information about both your internal state and the environment around you," Shams explained.

"So, it's like a bridge between the inner and outer worlds?" I queried.

"The core continuously updates the mind about the environment, sending cues that guide you toward behaviors ensuring balance, health, and harmony. But—and this is a significant 'but'—it expects the mind to listen," Shams clarified.

"And the mind doesn't always listen, does it?" I asked.

"Rarely," Shams replied. "The mind is like a recorder, a cocktail of memories, habits, beliefs, and attitudes. While the brain gathers messages from the environment through the senses, the mind processes them through its own filters. And these filters? They're often tainted by past experiences and personal perceptions."

"So, the information gets distorted?" I inquired.

"Precisely. Think of it this way: in an evolved and truly healthy individual, the mind and core exchange information freely. The core informs the mind of what is needed for well-being, and the mind translates these cues into actions. But in most cases, there is a check-valve between the two—a block that prevents smooth communication," Shams explained.

"A check-valve? What creates it?" I asked, intrigued.

"Rigid beliefs, unexamined habits, early indoctrination—everything the mind accumulates over time," Shams said. "Instead of being flexible and open, the mind calcifies, becoming a barrier that blocks the core's life-enhancing wisdom."

"What happens when this connection is blocked?" I pressed further.

"The mind starts operating on its own, cut off from the core," Shams answered. "The thoughts, decisions, and behaviors it generates are often selfish, colored by personal biases and devoid of concern for Nature or the environment. It's a half-baked understanding, shaped more by past programming than by present reality."

"And this misalignment affects the body too?" I asked, seeking clarity.

"Absolutely," Shams affirmed. "The mind is the primary communicator with the body, but when it's rigid, the messages it sends are incomplete and one-sided. Instead of fostering balance, it creates conflict—within the body and with the environment. That's where disease takes root."

"Is not rigidity of beliefs an ingredient for strong willpower, or are these two different things?" I questioned.

"That's an excellent question," Shams said thoughtfully. "At first glance, rigidity of beliefs might appear similar to strong willpower, but they are fundamentally different."

"How so? Aren't both about standing firm in something?" I asked, eager to understand.

"They may both involve firmness, but their roots and outcomes are entirely distinct," Shams explained. "Rigidity of beliefs comes from a place of fear, attachment, or a need for certainty. It is like a tree with shallow roots—it stands firm, but only because it refuses to bend. Eventually, a strong enough wind can uproot it."

"And strong willpower?" I inquired.

"Strong willpower, on the other hand, is like a deeply rooted tree that can sway with the wind yet remains unshaken at its core. It is flexible where needed but unyielding in its essence. This flexibility is what makes it resilient," Shams responded.

"So, rigidity is brittle, while willpower is adaptable?" I asked for confirmation.

"Exactly," Shams affirmed. "Rigidity locks you into a single way of thinking. It says, 'I know, and I refuse to consider anything else.' It might appear strong, but it creates tension within and conflict without."

"And willpower?" I probed further.

"True willpower is grounded in clarity and flexibility. It comes from alignment with your core. It gives you the strength to act with conviction, but without the blindness of stubbornness. Someone with true willpower can adapt to challenges, learn from experiences, and grow while staying true to their deeper principles," Shams clarified.

"So, rigidity and willpower are opposites?" I questioned to understand better.

"You could say rigidity is the enemy of willpower. Willpower thrives on an open, questioning mind, while rigidity shuts the door to growth. Rigidity is fear pretending to be strength—it resists change, making it fragile," Shams elaborated.

"How can someone move from rigidity to true willpower?" I inquired.

"By becoming self-aware. Start by asking yourself: 'Why do I believe this? Is it rooted in truth, or is it fear or habit?' The more you question and let go of what no longer serves you, the more flexible your mind becomes. And when your mind aligns with your core, true willpower emerges naturally," Shams advised.

"So, real willpower isn't about stubbornly holding on—it's about knowing when to hold on and when to let go?" I summarized.

"Perfectly put. True strength is not about resistance; it is about discernment. Flexibility is not weakness—it is wisdom in motion," Shams concluded.

"You mentioned earlier that rigidity blocks growth. How do we counteract that?" I asked.

"Through movement. Movement—whether physical, emotional, mental, or spiritual—is the antidote to stagnation. It is what allows us to break free from rigidity and explore new possibilities," Shams answered.

"Movement… like stretching?" I wondered aloud.

"Yes, stretching is a perfect example. Have you ever noticed how stretching leaves you feeling so refreshed and alive?" Shams inquired.

"I have, but I never stopped to wonder why," I replied.

"It's because when you stretch, you're expanding yourself—reaching beyond your usual boundaries into a new space. That act of reaching out, even into emptiness, creates a surge of energy," Shams explained.

"And this applies to more than just the body?" I questioned.

"Much more. Stretching is a metaphor for life. Physically, it energizes and relaxes you. Mentally, it builds confidence as you conquer new positions or perspectives. Emotionally and spiritually, it allows you to extend yourself toward others or the unseen force that sustains all life," Shams elucidated.

"So, movement across dimensions is essential for growth?" I sought clarification.

"Exactly. Whether it is stretching your body, challenging your beliefs, or reaching out to others, movement is what keeps life dynamic. It breaks the inertia of rigidity and allows you to connect with the core, the unseen, and the greater whole. It is this alignment that fosters true well-being—not just for the individual, but for the environment too," Shams affirmed.

"It sounds so simple, yet so profound," I observed.

"It is. Simplicity is often the hallmark of truth. The challenge lies in unlearning the rigidity and returning to the core's wisdom—a journey worth taking if you wish to live free of disease and in harmony with nature." Shams concluded.

As I walked away from my conversation with Shams, his words lingered. I realized that healing is not a destination; it is a journey—one that requires us to tune into the wisdom within ourselves. It is about listening to the body's instincts, drawing inspiration from the mind, trusting the gut's emotional resonance, and allowing the spirit to illuminate the way forward.

"Be supple like a Baby even with your
Beliefs for Growth & Evolution."

Being hard like a Dead Body
only reduces you to be a fodder
for the Lower organisms."

EPILOGUE

The Big Bang, often thought of as a mere explosion, was not just an eruption of cosmic proportions but an initiation, a divine spark designed to propel evolutionary growth. From the stardust to the complexity of humanity, this grand journey seems to suggest a profound purpose: for humans to ultimately become the guiding stars of creation and lead it toward its next evolutionary ascent.

Healing follows a similar pattern. It entails moving inward, from the periphery to the core. It is a shift from dis-ease, where chaos and imbalance dominate, to ease, where harmony and alignment are restored. The potential for this healing already exists within each of us. Just as the universe continues to expand, we can grow closer to our true selves, aligned with the light that guides all life.

This journey is shaped by the four interconnected dimensions of being:

The Physical Dimension safeguards us through our instincts.

The Mental Dimension guides us with inspiration.

The Emotional Dimension resonates with our gut feelings.

The Spiritual Dimension illuminates our path through revelation.

These dimensions work together to create balance, enabling us to find ease in our bodies, thoughts, emotions, and spirit. This harmony reflects the state of heaven often described in spiritual traditions—a place of ultimate freedom and peace. In a heavenly state, people are free to live and eat as they wish, yet they choose discipline. Why? Because their earthly lives of discipline and balance have prepared them for this freedom. They exist in a state of ease, not bound by chaos or indulgence, but enriched by harmony.

Contrast this with the people living in a state of hell, depicted as being chained. These chains symbolize the consequences of lives lived without discipline, where lessons of balance and harmony were ignored. Their chains bind them to a state of dis-ease, reflecting the turmoil they carry within.

Our own lives offer us the same choice. We can embrace discipline—not as a burden, but as a path to freedom. Discipline aligns us with the natural rhythms of life, allowing us to live with ease, unbound by the struggles that come from imbalance.

As you close these pages, remember that the answers you seek are already within you. Trust the process. Like the universe itself, you are designed to grow, evolve, and find your light.

ABOUT THE AUTHOR

Saleem Anwar is an entrepreneur with a global reach in the manufacturing sector, specializing in elastics for the shoe industry. He holds a degree in Mechanical Engineering and a Postgraduate degree in Mass Communication and Journalism. A lifelong learner, Saleem has expanded his expertise into the health field, holding certifications in Integrated Medicine, Indian classical acupuncture, and Yoga Training. He has also earned a diploma in Advanced Nutrition and Dietetics from Lincoln University, Malaysia.

Driven by a passion for understanding the deeper truths of health and wellness, Saleem has dedicated much of his study to exploring the connections between disease and lifestyle, with a particular focus on the impacts of modern healthcare systems.

With a profound interest in the balance between nature and human well-being, Saleem's passion extends to observing and addressing global challenges related to health, farming, and climate change. His reading pursuits encompass Classical Arabic and English Literature, Etymology, Evolutionary Biology, and Evolutionary Psychology.

Through his upcoming book *Disease to Ease*, Saleem presents a compelling exploration of the connection between distorted belief systems, aggressive attitudes, and the state of health. This work reflects his lifelong dedication to understanding and promoting holistic healing, offering readers a fresh perspective on achieving harmony and well-being.

www.ingramcontent.com/pod-product-compliance
Lightning Source LLC
Chambersburg PA
CBHW020342180726
47991CB00021B/2241